99 TRILLION HELPERS TO IMPROVE YOUR GUT HEALTH

HOW TO BOOST YOUR METABOLISM, PRODUCTIVITY, AND GENERAL WELLBEING IN AS LITTLE AS A MONTH WITHOUT POPPING ANY PILLS

DR P. K. SACITHARAN

CONTENTS

DISCLAIMER

This book does not claim to be a culmination of medical advice or meant to be used as replacement for any sort of medical treatment. The content is not authored by medical professionals and is only meant for educational and informational purposes only.

Please always consult your physician prior to getting started on or altering any dietary regimen or making any significant changes in your lifestyle, especially if you're dealing with chronic ailments like cardiovascular disorders, diabetes, hypertension and the likes.

Any prescription medicines must not be discontinued without professional advice. The author encourages the readers to gauge their condition and take suitable steps with due guidance from their physician at every step along the way.

INTRODUCTION

The gut is quite an extensive portion of the human body. It starts at the mouth and extends all the way down to the bottom-most tip of the large intestine. The esophagus, stomach, intestines, pancreas, gall bladder, and liver all come together to form the gut.

The gut is home to more than 100 billion bacteria. Surprisingly, for every 1 cell in the human body, there exist 10 microbes in the gut! Since the gut occupies such a crucial space, it is challenged with the most important functions as well. Every little progress in the body is heavily and directly influenced by gut health.

In the past few years, gut health has moved into the limelight with regard to a healthy lifestyle and dietary habits. It wasn't until the 1840s that the topic of gut microflora made its way in Western Literature. The bulk of study on this matter is concentrated in the late 1800s and early 1900s.

Today, gut microbiota is being extensively studied and discoveries are being made with each research study. Gut health has proven to be influential in all processes in the human body.

A healthy digestive system coupled with healthy microbiota is just the right tool for incredible immunity and overall good health. This is exactly what ***99 Trillion Helpers to Improve Gut Health*** aims to educate its readers on.

Why does gut health hold such unique importance?

> *"If there's one thing to know about the human body, it's this: the human body has a ringmaster. This ringmaster controls your digestion, your immunity, your brain, your weight, your health, and even your happiness. This ringmaster is the gut."* — Nancy Mure, Author

---

The gut is the direct recipient of anything we consume. Our diet, good or bad, has immediate repercussions on the digestive system and, consequently, the rest of the body.

In the maiden stage of my learning phase, I was very intrigued by the topic of gut health. I couldn't wrap my head around how one system can have such a profound effect on the rest of the body.

Prior to this, I believed that each system in the human body worked exclusively. Any shortcomings in one system remained limited to that system only. I was so wrong, and how!

Multiple research studies, in-depth knowledge, and years of experience have now compelled me to think otherwise. The truth is that any ups or downs in one part of the body create a ripple effect all over, especially when there is a malfunction in the gut.

Our body functions as one whole entity wherein all systems are interconnected. The digestive system, reproductive system, nervous system, respiratory system, cardiovascular system, and all other processes within our body are not mutually exclusive of each other.

This is why we lose our appetite or throw up when stressed, or we may have a temperature after a physical injury since our bodily systems all work in tandem with each other. They function interdependently to keep our body alive and well.

This explains why our gut holds such utmost importance in this regard. A strong gut comprises healthy microbiomes. Good bacteria and a host of immune cells work together to ward off infectious agents like harmful bacteria, viruses, and fungi.

Healthy gut microbiome results in smooth absorption of nutrients into the bloodstream, controlling blood sugar levels, good brain and heart health, and a stable state of mind.

Similarly, a weak gut causes a steady decline in mental health, productivity, and concentration along with poor physical health due to malabsorption of nutrients.

Often, symptoms like bloating, constipation, being underweight or overweight, and lethargy can all be traced back to poor gut health. Topical features like the quality of hair, skin, and nails are also largely influenced by our dietary choices and gut health.

In other words, a robust gut system is imperative to robust immunity.

The importance of gut health was realized decades ago but has only just begun to be implemented seriously. Right dietary choices, lifestyle habits, and mental health norms are now seeping into practice. These are nothing but attempts to keep our gut in shape so that our body and mind continue to function at their optimal capacity.

Mainstream medicine has surely progressed a lot in this aspect. We're now better aware of the importance of gut health than we used to be. While there is enough superficial knowledge floating around as to how and why one must prioritize gut health, it is now time to scratch beneath the surface.

Why should you listen to me, Dr. Pradeepkumar Sacitharan?

Gut health, like any other subject on health, should be learned about only from authoritative sources. Today, we are surrounded by umpteen channels to gain knowledge from but only a handful of them are truly reliable. *99 Trillion Helpers to Improve Gut Health* is, undoubtedly and unbiasedly, one of them.

My interest in gut health peaked at the very start of my career. Soon after obtaining a Ph.D. from the University of Oxford in Molecular and Cellular Medicine, I went on to train with world leaders in science and research.

Just like anyone else, I had my beginnings rooted in curiosity. I was quite intrigued by how our bodies perform at the cellular level. This further led me to research more on the gut microbiome, giving way to numerous peer-reviewed papers, books, and publications to my credit.

Currently, I run my own independent academic lab and am recognized as a respected consultant for global biotech companies. All my best experiences, knowledge, and understanding accumulated over the years have been carefully cherry-picked and compiled in this book.

What you hold right now is a condensed, information-rich, and error-free version of my thorough research work and personal studies. I have only dished out to you the cream of my career so that you can relish it and gain the same insight as me sans the hard work and sacrifices I underwent.

If you're an established expert on gut health, you might know plenty more than what is mentioned here, but you'll unquestionably second every bit of this book. Otherwise, you'll gain just the right information to pique your interest further on this subject.

Rest assured, you're in absolutely safe hands!

What can you expect from this book?

Through this book, I aim to address the dearth of deep, meaningful information on this subject. The goal of this book is to present to you an expertly crafted insight on gut health, a rich culmination of my knowledge, understanding, and experiences. I want to encourage you to take active steps toward a better, healthier future by safeguarding your gut.

This book carries just the right blend of basic lessons and detailed, authentic information without overwhelming you in any way. The language is precise, easy-to-grasp, and conveys technical aspects in straightforward terms. All technical words have been explained simply so that no reader stays devoid of any bit of matter conveyed in here.

99 Trillion Helpers to Improve Gut Health is the perfect choice of textbook for people who are keen on learning about what influences their health at the root. This includes young adults who're committed to maintaining a healthy gut, men and women beyond 40, teenagers, or anyone who wants to get familiar with this subject.

While this is not a medical textbook, the purpose here is to empower and educate you to make appropriate life choices for your betterment. You may be open to trying new dietary routines and lifestyle changes, but the first step is to recognize your symptoms, address them, and decide to take charge of your own health.

There is no mention of any devices or exercise patterns in this book, but you'll surely find an abundance of interesting, relevant information backed by thoroughly researched scientific sources and the latest studies. There are meal plans designed to go easy on your gut while not compromising your nutrient intake whatsoever.

In the following chapters, you'll receive a clear understanding of how the gut works, read the signs of your body, the right ways to supplement your nutrient intake, actionable tips to improve gut health, and healthy meal suggestions for the same. Moreover, you'll know how to look out for symptoms of poor gut health and fix them in time.

This book contains detailed strategies, in both dietary and non-dietary approaches, for optimizing gut health. This is a comprehensive guide for people from all walks of life and genders who wish to improve their gut performance.

I hope you walk away from this book armed with the right knowledge on gut health and the importance of preserving it, thereby paving the way to better overall physical and mental health.

See you on the inside!

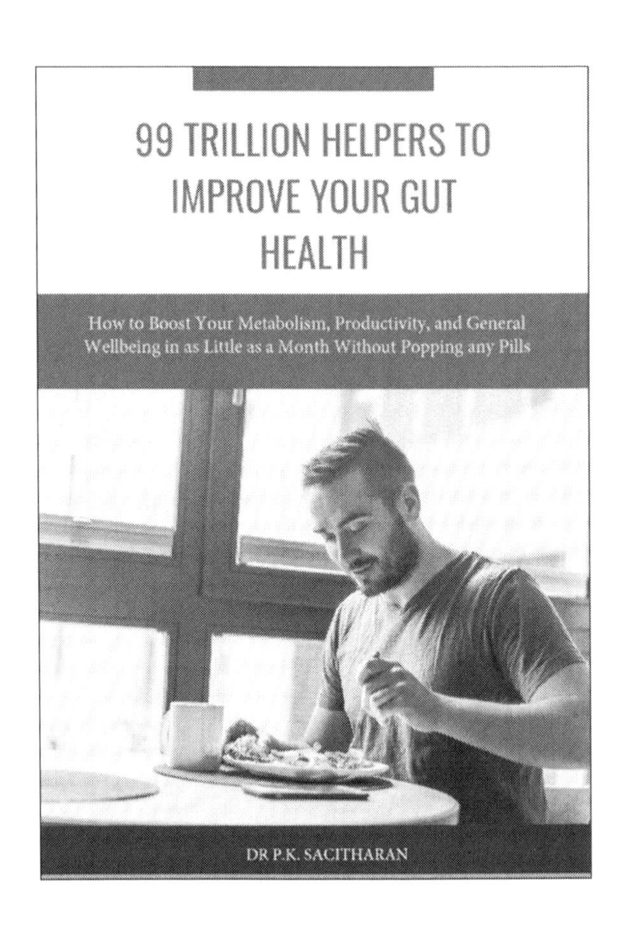

Scan the QR code to get your bonus recipe book:

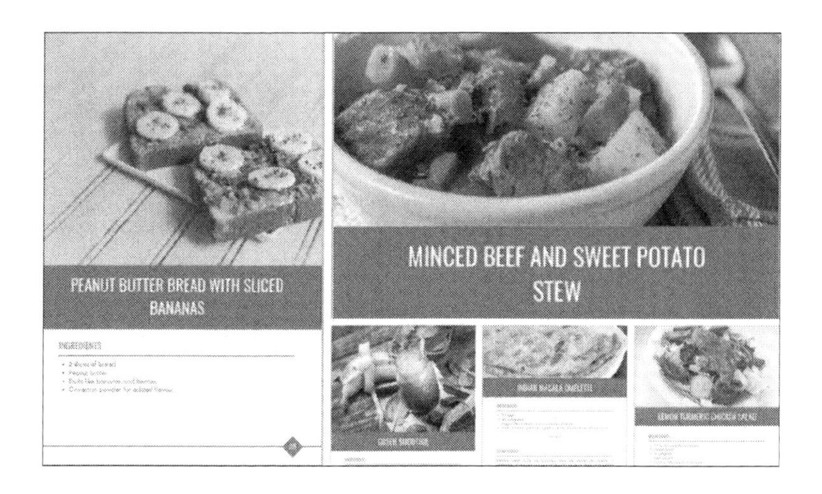

Join our Facebook group for more hints, tips, and like-minded people:

1

UNDERSTANDING YOUR GUT

No conversation about the gut is complete without mentioning digestion and metabolism, the primary roles of the gut organs. The series of hollow organs involved in absorbing and digesting food is collectively termed the "***gut.***"

A healthy gut includes a healthy stomach, intestines, pancreas, liver, and all other organs that are even remotely involved in the process of digestion. It wouldn't be an overstatement to say that the gut is the key to good overall health, including physical and mental well-being. [1]

Every cell, tissue, and organ in our body systems rely upon the gut to keep itself alive and functioning optimally. We all know that our body derives energy from the food we eat. This process is long and complicated.

It includes extracting the nutrients from the food, distributing them to the various parts of the body, and deriving energy from them. Digestion, metabolism, and assimilation all happen because of the gut. [2]

Our body can survive and function optimally solely because the gut breaks down the food we eat and chemically processes it, thereby deriving energy. These nutrients translate into power which smoothly enables daily physical activities.

UNDERSTANDING DIGESTION

Everything that we eat has a direct impact on our bodies. Our physical (and mental) health is an undeniable reflection of how well or poor our diet is. The process by which our diet is recognized and absorbed in our bodies is broadly termed "***digestion***."

A balanced diet is a healthy mixture of all key nutrients in regular, prescribed quantities. The 7 essential elements of nutrition—namely protein, fats, carbs, dietary fiber, minerals, vitamins, and water—need to be optimally present in our daily food intake for our body to function healthily.

These nutrients undergo a chemical breakdown in the digestive system for smoother absorption. Starting from the esophagus, the entire hollow passage that goes through the stomach right down to the anus is termed the "alimentary canal."

For better understanding, we always discuss digestion as a 6-step process. [3]

1. Ingestion:

Technically, ingestion is the first step of digestion, but the process is initiated a little before that. This step is the foremost and begins when the food enters our mouth.

As soon as you see the food and the aroma hits your nose, your digestive juice, namely the saliva, gets into action. Your mouth starts salivating and prepares itself to welcome the first bite of the delicious meal in your mouth.

Chewing with the teeth changes the texture of the food by manual degradation. Simultaneously, the saliva mixes with the food and converts it into a bolus that soon enters the stomach when we swallow it. This bolus passes down from the esophagus to the stomach. The rest of the process is involuntary until the last step, defecation.

2. Propulsion:

Propulsion happens when the food moves through the hollow organs of the gastrointestinal tract (GIT) by peristalsis (explained further in this chapter). The contents of the digestive tract keep propelling forward, thereby progressing in the process.

Without smooth propulsion, the organs of the GIT will not be able to receive the matter for digestion, resulting in improper absorption.

3. Mechanical or physical digestion:

Before undergoing chemical digestion, the food needs a thorough manual breakdown as well. It needs disintegration into smaller chunks for better absorption—the physical nature of the matter changes, but not its chemical composition. The first step of mechanical digestion, chewing, begins in the mouth.

Regardless of its original nature, the food is broken down and formed into a semi-solid bolus that is easier to digest. When the surface area and mobility of the smaller portions decrease, they move faster through the GIT.

Mechanical digestion is not just limited to the mouth. In fact, it takes place in all organs of the GI tract since the consumed matter keeps changing its form throughout the process. Squeezing, mixing, and changing forms from solid to liquid and back to solid fecal matter are all various forms of mechanical digestion.

4. Chemical digestion:

Mechanical digestion is not enough to get the food ready to be absorbed into the bloodstream. Therefore, enzymes and digestive juices get into action to degrade the complex molecules of the nutrient families into simpler molecules.

The protein is converted into simpler amino acids, the carbs become simple sugars, and so on. These vital nutrients, vitamins, and minerals further get distributed all over via the bloodstream, thereby translating into good physical well-being.

5. Absorption:

The food we eat is practically useless in the GIT until its nutrients are properly absorbed into the bloodstream. In other words, absorption is the most crucial step in the entire process of digestion.

Dietary deficiencies usually occur due to a dearth of certain nutrients in the diet. But deficiencies can also occur because of improper absorption within the digestive system and not due to a lack of nutrients in food.

Absorption begins in full force in the intestines, before which the process is mainly mechanical. The intestines are long, tubular, muscular organs that churn and re-churn the food to squeeze out the last bit of nutrient in it. The digestive enzymes from the pancreas and liver have a considerable role to play in this regard.

6. Defecation:

So far, your food has been squeezed and crushed and churned, both mechanically and chemically. Every usable bit of this consumed matter has been absorbed and assimilated into the bloodstream.

The leftover matter is now simply waiting to be discarded from the colon (large intestine) via the rectum through the anus. Ideally, an individual can hold their fecal matter voluntarily in the colon for 12–48 hours, although never advisable.

Defecation is a voluntary step, just like chewing and swallowing, in the entire digestive process that primarily consists of involuntary actions.

INTRODUCING REGULATORY MECHANISMS

The actions of all systems in the human body are intertwined, never exclusive. All systems in the human body have their independent functions. These systems have a set of specific organs designed to cater to those particular processes only. [4]

A malfunction within one system can cause a domino effect in other areas of physical well-being as well. Similarly, other crucial systems also extend some degree of interference in the digestive process—namely, the neural and hormonal controls.

The responsibility of these regulatory mechanisms is to maintain optimal conditions in the passage tubes for smooth digestion and absorption. This hormonal aid heavily catalyzes the digestive process resulting in a better chemical breakdown of the matter and faster assimilation into the bloodstream.

1. Neural control:

The muscular lining of the alimentary canal is full of nerve endings. These nerve endings function as sensory receptors detecting food's chemical and mechanical nature in the stomach and intestines.

Depending on the nature of its contents, these sensory receptors promote the secretion of respective enzymes to digest that particular type of food, like protein, fats, or carbs.

These receptors also sense physical needs such as how much the stomach needs to expand to accommodate its contents, how much more liquid or enzymes are needed to churn the same and to propel the matter forward through peristalsis once it has been digested.

Stimulation of these receptors is crucial to further the digestive process. Because of neural activity, the liver and pancreas secrete digestive juices to the intestines as soon as the latter receives digested contents down from the stomach.

The nerve endings in the muscular lining of the alimentary canal work in association with the central nervous system (CNS). Peristalsis is one such reflex action that stems from this function.

2. Hormonal control:

The digestive juices secreted throughout the entire course of digestion are nothing but a result of hormonal activity. Hormones cause the secretion of respective enzymes, which then carry out the core job.

To put it simply, think of the hormones as a checkpoint and the enzymes as the actual doer of the job. Whenever there is a need for enzymes, the hormones get into action and secrete the enzymes, which then carry out the job.

The joint activity of both hormones and enzymes is imperative to chemically degrade the food particles and move them from one organ to another.

The most crucial hormone of this process is present in the stomach, called gastrin. As the name suggests, this hormone causes the secretion of gastric acid by the inner mucosal lining of the stomach, which, in turn, breaks down the complex food matter into simple, digestible chunks.

HOW DOES FOOD MOVE THROUGH THE GI TRACT?

Understanding the GI tract:

Before we delve into how food is processed after it passes down the esophagus, let's understand the mechanism of the GI tract. The gastrointestinal tract comprises a series of organs that allow food to pass through them, each having a specific function.

Everything that we consume is churned in these organs serially, processed to extract as many nutrients as possible, and the remaining waste is discarded as fecal matter. Starting from the mouth, the GI tract consists of the esophagus, stomach, small and large intestines, and the anus. [5]

The only solid organs in the GI tract are the liver, pancreas, and gallbladder. These organs are hollow with an opening and exit that connect to the next organ in the series.

These solid organs secrete digestive juices called enzymes that catalyze the absorption of nutrients from the food into the bloodstream.

Understanding the passage of food:

The human body is full of miraculous networks, and the digestive system is the core of them all. Everything that we consume is received and processed by the digestive system. Just like all systems in our body function in tandem to keep us alive and well, so do the organs within each system.

As per the UNC, without the action of the enzymes, acids, and digestive juices of the GIT, one single meal would take about 2.3 billion years to get digested completely!

Speaking of the GI tract, the series of hollow organs work in sync to ensure the smooth passage of food right from the mouth down to the anus. Each organ undergoes contractions and relaxations to ease the course of the food mixture along the GI tract.

This phenomenon, called peristalsis, causes a wave-like motion in the organs, mixing everything thoroughly and propels its contents forward. [5]

As we know, our body and, therefore, all our systems are aligned vertically. The downward part of the organ relaxes while the upper part contracts, causing everything to move down to the next organ for the next step in the series.

The layer of muscle surrounding the walls of each organ of the GIT initiates peristalsis, which enables the smooth movement of the food in the downward direction. Due to this regular contraction and relaxation of muscles, the food we consume is churned well as it makes its way toward the end of the digestive canal.

Here is a brief outline of how each organ of the GIT participates in extracting the most from our food:

1. Mouth:

Did you know that the digestive process begins even *before* we eat? It sounds unbelievable, but your saliva gets the mouth ready to savor the first bite of your delicious dish right when you know it is time to sit down for a meal.

The smell and the sight of the food activate your enzymes and digestive juices, signaling that it is now time to get in action. This happens quite subconsciously.

Now you know why we suddenly feel pangs of hunger arising when we see an interesting dish or when the aroma from the kitchen hits our nose. It is your digestive system secreting digestive juices and preparing itself to receive some delicacies through your mouth and esophagus.

Once the food enters the mouth, the chewing action starts breaking it down both manually and chemically. Saliva has a big role to play in this regard. It breaks down the starch and sugars in the food and creates a soft lump in the mouth called the "bolus."

2. Esophagus:

The bolus then travels down to the esophagus, where it is pushed further by peristalsis. The bottom-most part of the esophagus is a ring-like structure called the lower esophageal sphincter that opens up to receive this bolus down from the throat into the stomach.

As soon as the food passes this checkpoint, the lower esophageal sphincter contracts again to prevent the contents of the stomach from coming up the throat. The muscular lining of the stomach stays strong to hold the contents of the stomach in its place.

Pregnant women often face extreme nausea and vomiting, especially in the first trimester. This happens due to the hormone "relaxin" secreted during pregnancy. It causes the muscular lining of the stomach to relax, thereby propelling its contents upward through the esophagus, making them gush out at the slightest discomfort.

3. Stomach:

The stomach is the first step of the digestive process where the food that we eat is introduced to the enzymes. We're still in the initial stage of the disintegration process.

By now, your food has been processed to some extent. It was disintegrated by chewing in the mouth, your saliva has also broken it down roughly, and now it has been passed down the esophagus into the stomach. Here is when the true process of digestion begins.

The inner lining of the stomach secretes strong enzymes and acids that mix with its contents and break it down further. Think of the stomach as a hollow space that is ready with strong acids, waiting to work upon anything that comes down your esophagus.

The churning of the stomach or feeling strong hunger pangs are nothing but the stomach acids at play. When your stomach is empty, the acids start eating up the inner lining of the stomach, and, hence, we feel burning and growling within our tummies!

4. Intestines:

Peristalsis causes the stomach to push down its matter to the intestines, where digestion continues. The small and large intestines are imperative to digestion. The small intestine is the first in the series, followed by the large intestine.

Both intestines are home to a broad range of gut flora and fauna, collectively termed as microbiota. This family of healthy bacteria is crucial to break down the matter chemically and catalyze digestion. [8]

Although the intestines don't secrete their own digestive juices, they churn the contents passed down from the stomach using the enzymes from the pancreas and bile from the liver. The liver is responsible for detoxifying the system and discarding all waste. [6]

Everything that we eat is now being processed along with liquids, enzymes, acids, and digestive juices. The matter enters the small intestine from the stomach as semi-solid and moves to the large intestine in an almost liquid state.

The colon or the large intestine is the final organ where the contents of the GIT are now squeezed and churned for the last time before being discarded. All possible nutrients have now been absorbed, and only nitrogenous, toxic waste is left over.

This indicates how crucial enzymes are. Without the enzymes, it would be impossible to extract nutrients from food and convert them into usable energy for everyday survival. We derive all our energy from food, and the gut enzymes have a major role to play in this conversion. [7]

QUICK RECAP

The GI tract is accurately designed to absorb all nutrition from the food. All organs of the digestive system, both hollow and solid, work in conjunction to extract as much nutrition from food as possible. This nutrition is then passed on through the bloodstream and distributed to the various sections of the body.

Digestion, absorption, and metabolism need to be catalyzed by acids and enzymes in the gut. These enzymes break down the complex material in the food, convert it into soluble, simple molecules, and absorb them in the body. Other neural and hormonal factors also influence the digestive process in the body.

The contents of the digestive system pass through all hollow organs of the GIT by peristalsis. Toward the end, all nutritional content is sucked out of it, and only nitrogenous, toxic waste is left over. This waste is then expelled through the anus.

2

A UNIVERSE OF MICROBES

Imagine you're playing this exciting, engaging video game where your character is aiding dozens of superheroes against an army of hundreds of unearthly villains. These villains are out to destroy the world and claim the Earth, and you're fighting them tooth and nail with a handful of mighty superheroes by your side.

A thrilling and decisive battle ensues, finally resulting in a clear winner: your army—the superheroes!

You have defeated the villains and are rejoicing with the heroes by your side, the onlookers celebrating your success. The game ends on your screen with pomp and a shower of the most delicate glitter, congratulating you on the astounding victory!

You are so proud of yourself, as you should be! After all, you're a winner!

The screen goes blank, and you're suddenly pulled back into the real world. Reality dawns on you as you look around your empty room and find yourself all alone. You're now dealing with the sinking feeling that follows after the end of an exciting game, a good book, or a long holiday.

What if I tell you that you've already been surrounded by similar superheroes all along?

In fact, you are never alone. An army of trillions of mighty and dynamic champions have been rooting for you and fighting for you all along. They are constantly backing you up against another army of bad guys.

Any guesses who they are?

These are your ***gut microbiota*** in action.

And the villains? They are the external bacteria, viruses, and various other infectious microorganisms that want to infiltrate your body and challenge your immunity.

DELVING DEEPER INTO THE FUNCTIONS OF THE GUT

Our body is a fascinating machine, capable of miraculous wonders. Each organ and system in the body works with a true purpose and is accurately designed to fulfill specific needs by functioning in association with the other systems.

The ***gut microbiome*** also plays a set role. There are umpteen microorganisms in the gut whose sole purpose is to keep your gut working in the most optimal fashion, which, in turn, keeps your health in the best shape. A positive domino effect ensues, reflecting in the functioning of other systems. [9]

When the gut can absorb and assimilate more nutrients from food, the other systems in the body like the nervous system, cardiovascular system, respiratory system, and reproductive system also function at their best. The gut and, hence, the gut microbiome fuel the rest of the body directly.

Our body is home to plenty of good bacteria present in our vital organs, scattered all over and within our bodies. Although 70% of the total microbiota in our body exists in the gut, the rest are present in other organs like the heart, lungs, placenta, mammary glands, skin, brain, and tissues like blood.

Within the gut, too, the microbiota is not equally distributed amongst the hollow organs of the gastrointestinal tract. The large intestine, for instance, has more significant microbial activity than the small intestine or the stomach. [10]

The gut microbiome survives on the nutrition gained from the human body. The gut microbiota are broadly classified into good and bad bacteria—***pathobionts***.

These beneficial and harmful bacteria are constantly at battle, the former always defeating the latter. However, sometimes the latter win due to external influences, such as foreign harmful bacteria or viruses, and causes sickness.

Drinking polluted water, coming into contact with a sick person, eating contaminated food, or any such reason can lead to infection in the body.

Infection is nothing but the result of harmful microorganisms infiltrating our system and providing aid to the bad bacteria in the gut. It is, therefore, essential to keep fueling the good bacteria in our system by strengthening our immunity with proper nutrition from food to help fight off infection if it occurs.

Gut heroes might sometimes fall short on energy and lose the fight against pathobionts and foreign infections. In such cases, doctors prescribe antibiotics to help deal with acute gut infections for immediate relief. These antibiotic medicines fight off harmful bacteria, sometimes even killing some good bacteria in the bargain. [11]

While antibiotics are the best short-term solution to cure an acute infection, they aren't always recommended for the long term. The gut microbiota can quickly become immune to antibiotics and can get resistant to small doses over time.

For instance, consider that your doctor asks you to take one tablet of antibiotics a day for 4 days in a row to cure your stomach infection. However, you end up missing 2 of the 4 days. Ideally, 4 days was crucial to uproot the disease at its core. However, now, the infection hasn't died but has only been weakened.

The harmful bacteria in the gut becomes immune to the small doses and ends up more robust than before. The chances are that these pathobionts will bounce back to health once the effects of the antibiotics wear off. [12]

The next time around, one tablet a day for 4 days will not be sufficient to get rid of them. You may need a higher and stronger dose to give the same results.

Consuming antibiotics can also mess up your gut ecosystem since it interferes with the natural mechanism in it.

Therefore, it is always important to consume antibiotics in specifically prescribed doses and never discontinue their use before that.

THE COMPOSITION OF THE GUT MICROBIOME

The terms ***"gut microbiome"*** and ***"gut microbiota"*** are pivotal to getting the hang of the gut functions and will often be used in this book. Let's understand them.

The gut microbiota is a collective term used to describe the microorganisms in the gut. It is a huge colony of both good and bad bacteria, viruses, eukaryotes, and all other types of microorganisms that influence our health. [13]

Microbiota is a family of microorganisms that differ in their genetic makeup and have varied functions per the organ or localization they survive in. For example, the gut microbiome has a specific set of tasks that may or may not be similar to the heart or skin microbiota.

On the other hand, the gut microbiome refers to the broader aspect of the gut ecosystem and environment.

It includes the entire microbiota with their genetic makeup and other factors like surrounding habitat, environmental conditions, and temperature.

Microbiota is an integral part of the microbiome regardless of the organ it is present in. Just like your video game wherein superheroes compete with villains to take control, so do the good bacteria constantly fight off the bad ones to keep your gut always working in the right order.

The intestinal functions primarily rely on gut heroes to take control over the gut villains, the pathobionts, and aid in the proper digestion of food. This constant opposition between the two types of gut microorganisms is crucial to ensure that the gut stays healthy without succumbing to the pathobionts.

An ideal condition is that healthy gut microorganisms stay dominant over the pathobionts, thereby establishing a powerful system with robust immunity. Such a condition is essential to the gut and, consequently, the human body to stay fit and healthy.

WHO AIDS THE GUT MICROBIOME?

Just like your character in the game aids the army of superheroes in the fight against the bad guys, a similar family of microorganisms stands in defense with the gut heroes against the pathobionts. And these are the ***probiotics.*** [14]

As the name suggests, probiotics work in favor of the good bacteria in the gut. These are additional soldiers that contribute to the superhero army, strengthening it further. Probiotics are not initially present in the gut but are taken in through diet.

A healthy dose of probiotics through a well-balanced diet is just the key to keep the army of your gut super-heroes consistently winning in the fight against the villains!

Speaking of probiotics, another class of plant-based nutrients called ***prebiotics*** is equally beneficial to the gut. Prebiotics fuel the existing good bacteria of the gut to perform better in keeping the gut environment actively functioning in the best manner. Probiotics, prebiotics, their functions, and their best food sources are discussed in detail further in this book.

Yogurt is the best source of probiotics to nourish the good bacteria in the gut. It contains bacteria Lactobacillus acidophilus and Lactobacillus casei that promote good bacteria quality and quantity. Yogurt is highly recommended to ease stomach discomfort during nausea, diarrhea, stomach aches, and constipation.

WHAT INFLUENCES THE GUT MICROBIOME?

The gut microbiome consists of trillions of microbes that encode about 3 million genes. These genes are responsible for carrying out the metabolic functions in the gut. For context, the entire human body, sans the gut microbiota, consists of only about 23,000 genes!

If we were to consider the gut microbiome when classifying the human body in the animal kingdom, humans would be more than 99% microbial!

Each individual has a different type of gut environment, determined by their lifestyle, diet, medications, and physical activity. About 1/3 of all individuals display the same gut microbiota, whereas 2/3 differ due to varying factors. Your gut microbiota can be strong or weak, depending on your lifestyle and diet. [15]

People with more physical activity, who rely on a healthy diet full of probiotics and prebiotics, and have regular circadian rhythms in terms of sleep and appetite, depict better gut health than the rest.

Several other factors determine the composition and strength of gut microbiota that we have no control over. Some of them are:

- Mode of birth (natural or C-section)
- Aging
- Genetics and heredity
- Gestational age (full-term or preterm birth)

For the longest time, scientists believed that the gut microbiome colony began developing before birth. But recent studies suggest that the child acquires their gut microbiome while being delivered through the vaginal canal.

The child is exposed to the mother's gut and vaginal microbiota, which dictates the growth of their own microbiome.

In a C-section delivery, the baby is exposed to the mother's skin microbiota and enters the external environment directly without receiving the vaginal microbiota. The lack of healthy exposure to the mother's gut microbiome is why Caesarean delivery and antibiotic use is not recommended, as they can alter this bacterial level in the infant. [16]

Further on, the mode of feeding the baby also influences the gut microbiome. Breast milk contains healthy lactic acid bacteria responsible for dictating the child's gut microbiome, which is not the same as when the baby feeds on formula milk.

Formula-fed babies sport a broader and much more comprehensive range of gut microbiome diversity. And the babies who rely on their mother's milk have a gut microbiome similar to their mother's.

By the time babies hit 2–3 years of age, their gut microbiome starts resembling that of an adult's, and this diversity stabilizes for the rest of their life with minor, seasonal variations.

QUICK RECAP

There are two exclusive classes of gut bacteria—the good bacteria and the pathobionts. They're each constantly at war with the other party. The side that wins decides the state of gut health.

Our diet plays a crucial role in building up the gut microbiota in both quantity and quality through probiotics and prebiotics, respectively.

Probiotics are good microorganisms themselves which increase the good gut microbiota in quantity. Best food sources of probiotics include yogurt, kimchi, pickles, and kefir. Probiotics increase microbiota in quantity.

Prebiotics are plant-based nutritional elements that strengthen the existing microbes in the gut and fuel them to perform better. Best food sources of prebiotics include whole grains, lentils, pulses, onions, and soybeans. Prebiotics increase microbiota in quality.

The gut microbiome is primarily influenced by several factors, especially in the early years of life. The diversity in the gut microbiota is mainly derived from the mother's gut and further by the diet and lifestyle habits adopted in early childhood.

3

WHY IS GUT HEALTH IMPORTANT?

The field of medicine in the 20th century witnessed many big leaps. Over time, however, a notion crept in that the body's various biological systems were highly compartmentalized and had little interconnection.

Today, it is well understood that this is not the case and that our vital systems not only communicate within the body but also influence each other's functions.

THE GUT AND THE OTHER ORGANS

Research has shown that the condition of one's gut can have a significant effect on the health and well-being of other organs, such as the brain and skin. It is also evident that besides physical effects, gut health has ramifications on psychological health as well.

Maintaining good gut health can enable the body to overcome panic attacks, stress, anxiety, depression, and even neurodevelopmental disorders such as hyperactivity and anxiety. [17]

In this chapter, we shall see how the gut can influence these factors and how it plays an active role in assisting the body to overcome these problems.

THE GUT-BRAIN CONNECTION

The connection between the gut and the brain is pretty intimate. We all have experienced at least a few moments where we feel the clear, distinct connection between our gut and brain. As mentioned before, the systems in our body don't work exclusively from each other. [19]

Any malfunction in one system does reflect in the functioning of the others. Similarly, any stress or happiness in the brain has a simultaneous effect on gut health as well. When the mind is tense, so is the gut.

We often lose our appetite before a big day, event, important interview, or exam. Our mind is so occupied with stress that there's no scope to consider eating. And once we're through the big event our stomachs start grumbling with pangs of hunger!

A psychological hack is to chew gum just before taking an important exam or appearing for an interview. This signals to your subconscious brain that because you're eating your mind and body are not really in danger, and therefore there's no need to panic. Your mind is tricked into calming down, instead of stressing, which helps you to concentrate better on the task at hand.

Some of these symptoms include constant nausea, stomach twinges and aches, frequent vomiting or diarrhea, losing one's appetite, or not being able to retain food for long. [18]

On the other hand, being happy and content translates into a healthy appetite and smooth digestive processing. This indicates that the mind has a very strong hold over our gut health.

Casual phrases like "follow your gut," "gut-wrenching," "butterflies in your stomach," or "pit of the stomach" all stem from this intimate and very real connection between the gut and the brain.

This connection is clinically termed the ***"gut-brain axis."***

What is the gut-brain axis?

The gut-brain axis refers to the bidirectional communication between the enteric and central nervous systems and how the two systems influence each other. It explains how cognitive and emotional health is connected with peripheral intestinal functions. [20]

Anatomically speaking, the gut is connected to the brain through the vagus nerve of the autonomic nervous system. It is a crucial component responsible for involuntary body functions such as breathing, swallowing, and food digestion.

The gut microbiota with its tens and trillions of organisms, most of which live in the large intestine, are in constant cross-talk with each other affecting not only physical but also mental health. This actually goes both ways with mental strain such as stress and anxiety having a detrimental effect on gut health.

How does it work?

As discussed before, the gut is home to trillions of microbes that we acquire from the birthing canal during the delivery process and also in the first few years of life. These microbes, including all microbiota from all internal organs, can have a cumulative weight of up to 2.7 kg, but they remain obscured from the naked eye due to their miniscule size.

The enteric nervous system, or the digestive nervous system, itself has about 100 million nerve cells distributed throughout the gastrointestinal tract. These nerve cells are directly connected to the brain's ***"fight or flight"*** response system and the ***"rest and digest"*** mode. These responses send signals in stressful situations through the ***sympathetic and parasympathetic*** nervous systems.

When the mind is placed under extremely stressful situations, it either goes into "fight" mode or "flight" mode, which is running away from the danger. This is called the "fight or flight" response, which is initiated by the sympathetic nervous system.
The fight or flight response is often followed by the "rest and digest" mode which is activated by the parasympathetic nervous system. In the latter stage, the body cools down from the urgency after the effects of the danger has passed.

The gut, on the other hand, relies on neurotransmitters and immune cells to transmit messages to the brain. It hosts millions of immune cells in addition to microbes. These immune cells examine the GI tract for any abnormalities such as GI infections, inflammation, inadequate blood flow, or bloated stomach and relay this information to the brain.

Microbes use neurotransmitters as messengers to the brain. The beneficial bacteria Lactobacillus rhamnosus, for instance, uses the neurotransmitter gamma-aminobutyric acid (GABA) to modulate brain activity and relieve anxiety. [21]

Through specific diets, we can alter bacteria levels in the gut and treat mental health issues such as panic attacks, stress, anxiety, depression, autism, and hyper-activity.

In addition to treating the above issues, good gut bacteria can promote better mental health by secreting beneficial chemicals such as serotonin and butyrate. Serotonin is a neurotransmitter that regulates happiness levels, whereas butyrate is responsible for good gut health.

The good gut bacteria produce butyrate by breaking down nutrition from plant sources like veggies, fruits, legumes, nuts, whole grains, and seeds. Butyrate is an essential chemical for maintaining the cells in the gut lining. It also reduces inflammation, improves overall mood, and helps the brain create new brain cells. [22]

The above examples make it abundantly clear that the gut and brain are heavily intertwined. Negative emotions such as fear, anger, sadness, and anxiety can have an adverse effect on gut health, even resulting in conditions such as irritable bowel syndrome (IBS) in extreme cases.

However, this is a two-way street. Just like the state of our mind dictates our gut health, our gut health also has a direct influence on our mind. As per the latest research, prolonged gut issues like IBS, inflammation, or any other changes in the gut microbiome result in severe mental health disorders like Parkinson's disorder, anxiety, or depression.

The amazing benefits of having 100 trillion gut bacteria at our disposal are not limited to just changes in mental health. In addition to influencing mental health, a healthy gut can promote a fitter body too. The gut microbiota contains many beneficial bacteria that can improve the health and overall shape of a body.

If the mind is going through stress, the gut follows suit. Tragic events like divorce, death of a loved one, witnessing accidents involving blood and gore, or any trauma that deeply impacts the mind, impact the gut as well. It causes nausea, vomiting, loss of appetite, weight loss, or diarrhea since the gut is just as stressed as the mind.

THE WEIGHT-GUT CONNECTION

Just like there's a gut-brain axis, there's a weight-gut axis too. The gut plays an integral role in absorbing nutrients from the food and assimilating them into the bloodstream to be distributed to the various organs in our body.

Therefore, there is a close connection between gut health and the physical condition of our bodies. Being fat, thin, lean, or fit are all reliant on how well the gut is performing.

Losing or gaining weight are also done by altering the function of the gut microbiome.

This is especially true for a diverse microbiota. The different bacteria that colonize the colon perform different functions.

The more diverse this group, the better our metabolism, which ultimately keeps the weight in check. This may be why some people do not put on weight despite having a greater-than-average appetite. [22]

How does it work?

There is no gut bacterium that can cause weight loss directly. Instead, it is the cascading effects of having the right microbiome that translates into weight loss benefits.

According to studies, lean people had 70% more gut bacteria and, therefore, an increased gut microbiome diversity than their overweight counterparts. In fact, researchers claimed that by just examining the gut microbiota, they would be able to tell whether a person was lean or overweight.

As our understanding of the gut microbiota increases, we are able to identify more and more beneficial bacteria that carry out specific tasks and contribute to slimmer waistlines. Let us consider a few examples of gut bacteria.

- Christensenella minuta

Christensenella is a good gut bacterium that has recently become popular due to its weight control effects. Whether you have it or not will most likely be determined by your genetic makeup. If your family has it, you are more likely to have it.

Research found that although 96% of samples had Christensenella, leaner people had a significantly higher number in their gut compared to obese people. They believe that understanding the relationship between this bacterium and obesity could help prevent obesity in the world at large, considering that obesity is now a global epidemic.

- Akkermansia muciniphila

Another example is that of Akkermansia muciniphila. It feeds on the mucus of the gut lining, enabling an increased production, ultimately strengthening the intestinal barrier. A weaker gut lining is associated with obesity. This bacterium also produces acetate, which helps the body regulate its fat stores and appetite, controlling weight.

There are two ways to increase A. muciniphila levels: a balanced diet and physical workouts. Adding variety to your diet—various fruits, vegetables, whole grains, etc. —helps to increase the biodiversity in the gut and promote A. muciniphila production. Similarly, a good workout can do wonders for the gut's biodiversity.

As per an Irish study conducted on male rugby players, individuals who exercised more often sported a wider array of microbes than those who didn't. The players who worked out more often also had higher levels of A. muciniphila which has been proven to bring down body fat and flab. This shows that the good bacteria level in the gut increases with higher physical activity and also promotes a leaner, fitter, and stronger body.

- Helicobacter pylori

Helicobacter pylori or, as it is more commonly known, "H. pylori" is an ideal example of how cascading effects of various bacteria can cause weight loss. H. pylori is actually responsible for peptic ulcers and cancers, but this infection does not occur in most people. When it does, the doctor will prescribe antibiotics as treatment.

Antibiotics have brought down H. pylori cases to 50% of their original rates, but there are certain negative effects of such a reduction. H. pylori restricts the production of ghrelin, a hunger hormone, in the stomach.

This hormone makes us feel hungry and prompts us to eat. On eating, H. pylori reduces the production of ghrelin, curbing hunger pangs. In the absence of H. pylori, ghrelin levels do not diminish, making us eat more than necessary. Leptin, on the other hand, is the hormone that suppresses our appetite as soon as we are full.

The hormones ghrelin and leptin induce and suppress hunger respectively. An imbalance in the secretion of these hormones can cause a fluctuation in appetite levels thereby directly promoting unhealthy weight loss or weight gain.

THE SKIN-GUT CONNECTION

Similar to the brain and weight, the gut influences skin health too, termed the "skin-gut axis." The skin is the largest organ of our body. On a daily basis, it is exposed to many physical, chemical, and bacterial challenges in the environment. It defends the internal organs, and the body at large, against these challenges.

What is the skin-gut axis?

In addition to the above-mentioned external challenges, the skin can indicate issues in the internal systems as well. It manifests these internal issues through a variety of different symptoms, making us aware of an internal struggle and what could be causing it. [23]

Any unfavorable changes in the gut microbiome present on the skin in the form of rashes, boils, reduced skin cell turnover, and other skin conditions such as dermatitis, rosacea, and acne. This relationship between the gut and the skin is known as the skin-gut axis.

Scientists have been researching and exploring the connection between the gut and skin since as far back as the 1930s. In 1961, for example, a study revealed that 80 percent of 300 acne patients showed significant improvement when treated with probiotics.

How does it work?

The digestive tract is actually much larger than is apparent from its compact size. Overall, it has an area of 320–430 square meters, making it one of the largest interfaces between the human body and the environment.

The trillions of bacteria that live in the gut usually maintain homeostasis throughout the body. As we have already learned, they help us maintain physical and mental health and keep our bodies in the best shape.

Acting as a barrier between the digestive tract and circulation, the gut microbiome breaks down the food into nutrients that are then absorbed into the bloodstream and delivered to their appropriate destinations.

When certain allergic foods or medication, alcohol, antibiotics, artificial coloring, harmful bacteria, etc. cause gut irritation/inflammation, the immune system supercharges and gets ready to fend off the gut from invasion.

The gut lining may become thinner than usual, causing some bacteria/microbes to enter circulation. This activates the immune system further, and the effects are manifested in the form of skin ailments and inflammation in various other body parts.

One of the crucial aspects of dealing with stubborn acne and dull skin is to stay hydrated. Keeping yourself hydrated is the key to flushing out toxic waste from the gut and out of the body which then results in clear, glowing, supple skin.

Dysbiosis in the gut:

At times, our gut fails to perform to its best. Certain conditions lead to sluggish movements in the gut that need to be dealt with medically. This is often caused by external factors such as antibiotics, acute infections, or poor diet which can result in an unbalanced gut microbiome.

Such an unbalanced state is known as dysbiosis and can have a huge impact on other bodily functions. At times, the effects of dysbiosis are easily visible, such as in the case of cow milk allergy in toddlers. The presence/absence of a gut bacterium, Anaerostipes caccae, can prevent/cause an allergic reaction to cow milk and certain other foods.

In other cases, the link between skin issues and gut health may not be as obvious and may need further investigation. Over the years, connections have been discovered between various other skin conditions and gut health. Let us take a look at some of these popular correlations.

1. Acne:

Acne is much more prevalent in western countries. About 85% of people between the ages of 12–25 suffer from it. Experts have linked the high occurrences of acne in western countries to the high glycemic load of carbohydrates in their diet.

This diet promotes the formation of insulin-like growth factor (IGF-1). Greater levels of IGF-1 cause intense acne formation.

2. Dermatitis:

An immune reaction against gluten consumption is known as celiac disease. This disease can trigger dermatitis herpetiformis in the skin which shows up in 10 to 15% of celiac disease patients.

When patients with celiac disease consume gluten, their intestine creates immunoglobulin A (IgA) antibodies. When these antibodies bind with epidermal transglutaminase protein, they lead to dermatitis.

3. Rosacea:

Rosacea is a condition that causes red, pus-filled bumps on the facial skin. A study showed that small intestinal bacterial overgrowth (SIBO) is 10 times more likely to appear in patients suffering from rosacea. On treating SIBO, the skin cleared in almost all patients.

More and more connections are being made between physical ailments and gut conditions with every new study. Our attitude, weight, skin health, sleep quality, stress response, mood, immunity, and metabolism are all influenced by gut health.

There is no dissenting opinion among experts that a thriving gut considerably improves our quality of life in all spheres. Improving gut health must, therefore, be a top priority.

QUICK RECAP

The gut is pivotal to the uninterrupted operation of the rest of the vital systems in our body. Hence, there is a direct correlation between gut health and mental health, the skin, and our body weight.

This direct correlation is made apparent through the works of certain specific bacteria. This also shows how there is an interconnection between gut health and the health of the various other systems in our body.

It is crucial for the gut to stay healthy in order to ensure the smooth working of the rest of the body. Any malfunction in the gut ultimately shows up in visible forms like unhealthy weight loss or weight gain, dry and patchy skin, and declining mental health.

Our mental health is closely influenced by our gut health. Stressful situations, trauma, and anxiety can have direct, immediate impacts on the gut resulting in vomiting, diarrhea, and weight loss.

4

THE GUT FEELING—SYMPTOMS OF POOR GUT HEALTH

With regard to both location and function, the gut is at the core of the human body. Any malfunction in any part of the body has a direct effect on gut health. Similarly, a defect in the smooth operation of the gut also greatly influences the rest of the anatomy.

Sometimes, owing to certain reasons, our gut health is compromised. It could be because of generic conditions like having an upset stomach, eating stale food, indigestion, the impact of medications, dehydration, or mental health issues like stress and anxiety.

Good gut health is the key to good overall health. Initially, scientists and the general public believed that the symptoms of an unhealthy gut only meant indigestion, bloating, and diarrhea. Today, research studies show that the symptoms of poor gut health are linked to a host of other disorders.

As Hippocrates, the father of modern medicine, rightly claimed, ***"All diseases begin in the gut."***

The initiation of all diseases in the body can be traced back to a core malfunction in the gut. Indigestion, improper metabolism, and a leaky gut are the first direct signs of something wrong occurring within the system.

The more indirect signs of declining gut health include disorders of other organs like diabetes and obesity, which we usually don't associate with a gut disorder at all! Other aspects of overall well-being like stable mood, hormonal balance, strong immunity, supple skin, good brain health, and physical energy are all negatively affected if there is something wrong in the gut.

Chronic conditions like diabetes, obesity, chronic fatigue syndrome, specific nutrient deficiencies, and even mental health disorders like depression can all be traced back to a faulty gut.

The gut is quite robust. It is full of acids, enzymes, and digestive juices that can fend off any form of foreign infection. The immune system aggressively backs up the gut since the body knows that the gut houses the most critical element crucial for survival, the fuel for the body, the source of all nutrition: food.

However, often due to improper dietary habits and lack of good immunity, the gut loses the fight against foreign microorganisms and falls prey to such infection. When that happens, the symptoms of poor gut health start manifesting themselves in different ways.

WHAT GIVES RISE TO POOR GUT HEALTH?

The strength of the gut is its microbiome. The more diverse the gut microbiota, the better it is for our gut health. Our gut microbiota starts gaining diversity right at birth. The baby absorbs the mother's microbiome while passing through the vagina during childbirth and later via her breast milk.

Nowadays, due to the increased frequency of C-section births and young babies thriving on formula milk, we're witnessing less and less diversity in people's gut microbiome. And the less diverse the microbiota is, the more susceptible the person will be to a weak gut in their later years.

A robust gut is synonymous with strong immunity and vice versa. There is a stark difference in immune tolerance levels in children who grew up in sheltered homes as opposed to those who had extremely rough beginnings in life.

The former set of children are usually not exposed to unsupervised meals, a flexible diet, or even dirt, unlike the latter set, who develop quite a strong resistance to infections due to their lifestyle habits.

Generally, western societies and developed nations usually have a weaker gut than their counterparts in third-world countries or less-developed areas of the world for the same reason.

The key to building a good immunity in young children is to let your child go a bit wild with their diet and playing habits in their early years, obviously under supervised conditions. [27]

If you have family in developing nations in the world and often fly down to meet them, you might have noticed your gut is unable to digest the local food and water there. Diarrhea, nausea, and stomach aches become a common occurrence on such trips.

This happens because your gut is accustomed to a limited range of bacterial diversity and cannot keep up with the wide range of bacteria in the food, air, and water in such countries which the local citizens have no problem consuming!

This is not a problem for people moving from developing nations to western societies since their gut is already strong and habituated to much more diverse microbiota than what is available here.

Pediatricians often encourage parents to let their children outdoors to play in the dirt, run around barefoot in parks, or get cozy with pets. It helps build a strong immunity for the child and, consequently, a robust gut microbiome in their adult years.

There can be various reasons leading to malfunctions in the gut, but the symptoms are common and often rooted in similar causes. The symptoms of a faulty gut can be broadly classified into 3 categories: inflammation, autoimmune conditions, and poor nutrient absorption.

1. Inflammation:

Inflammation is the most common and the most obvious consequence of poor gut health. All general health issues of the gut like diarrhea, stomach ache, bloating, and nausea stem from a weak gut.

This condition is characterized by a slight reddening or swelling of the affected area, often accompanied by pain. This is the immune system's response to an irritant or a foreign particle in the body. The white blood cells, WBCs, rush to the irritated area and cluster together to form a protective sheath. This sensitivity is termed inflammation.

The WBCs are also known as the "soldiers of the body." Multiple types of cells make up the immune system, but the WBCs are the core strength of this system. Abnormally high levels of WBCs in the blood indicate an infection in the body.

Inflammatory bowel disorder or IBD is one of the most common inflammatory responses of the immune system. Stomach ulcers caused by celiac disease, gluten intolerance, ulcerative colitis, and Crohn's disease all happen due to inflammation. (Discussed below in detail.)

While inflammation can be tricky to spot visibly, there are some direct indications of it. For example, ulcerative colitis affects the large intestine and makes it difficult to absorb nutrients from food. Improper nutrient absorption can also lead to a sudden, unexplainable weight loss. [31]

There are many more direct and indirect consequences of inflammation in the gut. Some of them are listed below:

- Chronic fatigue and lethargy
- Brain fog
- Insomnia
- Skin diseases like psoriasis
- Hormonal imbalances

An inflamed gut cannot process sugar and store it in the liver, leading to frequent cravings for sugary foods and empty calories. An unhealthy weight gain is inevitable if one gives in to these cravings. In other words, inflammation in the gut can cause sudden weight loss or weight gain depending on other factors like lifestyle and dietary habits.

2. Autoimmune conditions:

The immune system is designed by nature to tackle all kinds of threats and infections from the outside world. It is a sturdy system, tough enough to take on all types of challenges without your conscious mind even realizing it. [28]

However, if your surroundings are too clean and there is practically no threat to your body even from food or water, the immune system becomes, in simple terms, "jobless."

Such a robustly designed system now finds itself incapable of providing support to your body since there is no particular need for the same. Hence, this immune system now turns upon itself and starts attacking cells within the body.

Due to lack of exposure to harmful substances, the system is now hurting its own body in the bargain. This also explains why autoimmune conditions are more prevalent now than ever, especially in first-world globally developed countries.

This is one of the many probable causes of autoimmune disorders. The concept of autoimmune conditions is relatively new. In the last century, such diseases were grouped together under a common category called "***autoimmune disorders***."

Health researchers worldwide are still engaged in an ongoing debate about what constitutes a proper definition of this term and the root cause of autoimmunity in the body.

Although it is not yet possible to pinpoint the exact reasons that give rise to autoimmune conditions, some pivotal factors help define them. Diet and lifestyle habits play a significant role in this regard. Foods that are high in fat and processed sugar are known to be closely linked to autoimmune conditions.

Diseases like hay fever, allergy to pollen, joint pain, and various other food allergies are more common in the western developed nations than in the rest of the world. The reason boils down to a generally sanitized and safe environment with little to no pollution or contamination.
As globalization is on the rise, the occurrence of autoimmune conditions in the world is also escalating.

Now that we know the general causes of autoimmune disorders, let's steer ourselves back to our core subject: poor gut health. While many autoimmune responses can occur for various reasons, let's discuss some conditions that directly affect the gut.

- <u>Type 1 diabetes:</u>

Insulin, the hormone required to break down and digest sugar, is produced in the B-islet cells of the pancreas. Without insulin, the body cannot synthesize blood sugar, leading to dangerously high sugar levels.

In type 1 diabetes, the immune system begins attacking these insulin-producing cells, which causes a severe dearth of insulin in the body. Unlike type 2 diabetes that usually occurs in older adults *(**adult-onset diabetes**)*, this condition is mainly prevalent in young people. It is, therefore, also called ***juvenile diabetes.***

- Celiac disease:

This condition causes the gut to become overly sensitive to gluten. Gluten is a protein widely present in starchy foods, grains, and cereals like wheat, rye, etc. When gluten particles enter the small intestine, the gut cannot process them which results in immediate inflammation of its inner lining.

Gluten sensitivity, a much more common condition than celiac disease, is a milder version of gluten intolerance but has similar symptoms like diarrhea and stomach aches.

- Inflammatory bowel disease (IBD):

IBD is characterized by inflammation of the inner lining of the intestinal walls. There are two types of IBD: Crohn's disease and ulcerative colitis. The former can affect any part of the GIT, while the latter causes inflammation in only the large intestine.

But what exactly goes wrong in the gut that triggers such autoimmune responses?

As we already know, the gut houses a complex community of micro-organisms collectively known as the gut microbiota. These microorganisms play a huge role in the digestion and metabolism of food and are kept sealed well within the hollow organs of the GIT.

However, due to malfunctioning in the gut or sometimes due to the gut lining giving way, some microbiota can seep into the bloodstream, often infiltrating nearby organs. This breach of the gut lining, known as a ***leaky gut***, is not a common occurrence but is not entirely impossible. (Leaky gut is discussed in detail later in the book.) [33]

A recent research study conducted by Dr. Martin Kriegel at Yale demonstrated that the microbes escaping the gut organs and moving into the bloodstream have a massive role in giving rise to autoimmune responses in the body. [34]

Summing it up, one of the possible reasons for an autoimmune response in the body could be a leaky and weakened gut.

Other symptoms of autoimmune conditions include...

> ... food intolerance and allergies since the gut is unable to metabolize certain foods
> ... joint pain

... hormonal imbalances
... nutrient deficiencies due to malabsorption of food.

3. Poor nutrient absorption:

Absorption is a crucial step in the digestive process that lays the foundation for further efforts like distribution and assimilation. Poor nutrient absorption is one of the most significant drawbacks of having a malfunctioning gut.

Despite there being no shortage of nutrients in the diet, the body still faces nutrient deficiencies since the gut cannot absorb them well.

Some conditions that point toward nutrient deficiencies include:

- Thinning, dry hair
- Dry, patchy skin
- Chronic fatigue

However, it is essential to check if you're consuming a well-balanced diet and having your meals on time. If the nutrient deficiencies still exist, then the possibility of faulty nutrient absorption due to improper gut function can be considered.

Poor nutrient absorption may also lead to unintentional and sudden weight loss or weight gain. Since the body cannot store fat and regulate blood sugar levels, there may be a sudden urge to overeat, causing weight gain. [36]

Similarly, lack of nutrient absorption can result in SIBO, leading to unhealthy weight loss and weakness over time. Since the gut is unable to process and store glucose in the liver under such circumstances, it "leaks" out into the bloodstream often leading to itchy skin and dry patches.

The gut microbiota now starts to crave sugar which creates an unhealthy urge for consuming the same. If one gives in to this craving, it only fuels the bad bacteria in the gut without addressing the real issue, thereby only continuing this vicious cycle.

QUICK RECAP

Poor gut health is the leading cause of all other disorders that occur in our bodies. Inflammation, autoimmune responses, and poor nutrient absorption are the most apparent symptoms of gut malfunction. This is your body's way of drawing your attention to something that needs fixing within the body.

Addressing poor gut health is the first step to maintain good overall health. Multiple factors go into play when setting gut health right. The key to a strong gut is implementing the right strategies of a balanced diet, a solid exercise regimen, and some profound lifestyle changes that promote healthy well-being in the long run.

5

EAT PREBIOTICS FOR YOUR GUT

With all its organs and systems, our entire body thrives on the nutrition that we derive from our food. A well-balanced diet contains all nourishment that replenishes the strength of each organ of the body in all aspects.

These varied nutritional elements are scattered in our food items. Just to brush up on our knowledge, here are some essential elements of nutrition and the respective roles they play in our bodies.

- **Proteins:**

Also known as the ***body's building blocks***, proteins are essential to repair the wear and tear of our system.

Growing children require an abundance of protein in their diet since their body is building its way up.

Adults, on the other hand, only need protein to keep their grown-up bodies in shape. Our hair, skin, and nails are majorly made up of protein. The digestive process breaks down protein into simpler amino acids, which then perform various functions in respective locations in the body.

The daily protein requirement for children is about 1.5 g per 1 kg body weight, while adults need just about 1 g per 1 kg of their body weight. Therefore, a child weighing 12 kg needs 18 g protein, and an adult weighing 70 kg needs 70 g protein per day.

- **Carbohydrates:**

Commonly known as carbs, these are abundantly present in almost all our food items. All types of cereals, grains, bread, and pulses contain carbs. Chemically speaking, carbohydrates are complex clusters made up of simple sugars crucial for survival.

When consumed in excess, carbs get stored in the body for later use if the need arises. Excess carbohydrate deposits in the body lead to unhealthy weight gain over time.

Glucose, or blood sugar, is a simple sugar and a significant component of complex carbs. It is the primary energy source for the brain, blood, and various other cells and tissues in the body.

The brain is encapsulated in a special covering called the blood-brain barrier that isolates it from the bloodstream and the rest of the body. No element, except glucose, can breach this barrier.
When we feel dizzy or light-headed, the first thing to do is to lie down and eat something sweet containing glucose. Glucose immediately gets absorbed and penetrates the blood-brain barrier, and provides much-needed nourishment to the brain.

- **Fats:**

Dietary fats are a major source of energy for our system, second only to carbs. In the case of excess consumption of fats, they're stored in the body and put away for later use. But when unhealthy fats are consumed in excess, they start interfering with the smooth functioning of the body.

Contrary to popular belief that fats need to be consumed sparingly, fats should make up about 30% of our total dietary intake. A healthy dose of sufficient dietary fats in our system is imperative to keep our vital organs going.

Broadly speaking, 3 types of fats are abundantly available in our food: ***saturated, unsaturated, and trans fats***. Of these 3 types, only unsaturated fats are healthy, while the other 2 are best avoided. Butter, cheese, red meat, and various oils are rich in saturated and trans fats and, hence, should be consumed sparingly.

There are two classes of vitamins: water-soluble (B and C) and fat-soluble (A, D, E, and K). When there is a shortage of fat in our system, our body cannot absorb and metabolize the fat-soluble vitamins, thereby leading to a serious deficiency of the same.

WHAT ARE PREBIOTICS?

Just like the different body parts need some standard elements of nutrition to thrive upon, the gut microbiota also needs some nourishment from food. And the primary source of strength for the complex community of microorganisms residing in the gut is prebiotics. [38]

Prebiotics are plant-based fibers that work to reinforce the existing microbes in the gut and give them the required nourishment to improve their performance by several notches.

The gut doesn't directly digest them. Hence, they move to the lower portions of the GIT, wherein they work as a source of nourishment for the good gut bacteria and easing bowel movements. [45]

The prebiotic fibers are just what the gut needs to keep functioning smoothly. Fibers are an important class of nutrients that do impart nutrition but cannot be stored in the body for emergency purposes. Any excess fiber in the system is immediately expelled. [39]

Fibers, therefore, have a different function. They act as a binding agent that helps propel the contents of the gut forward. They bulk up the fecal matter for easy passage of the same via the anus. Constipation is the first symptom of a lack of fiber in the diet.

Largely speaking, fiber mainly performs in the gut. It strengthens the microbiota, smooths the digestive and metabolic processes, and keeps you satiated for long. Therefore, the gut suffers largely if you don't include enough prebiotic fiber in your diet. [40]

Quickly brushing up on the magical effects of prebiotic fiber:

- Strengthens the gut microbiota and enables them to fend off foreign infections
- Bulks up the fecal matter to ease constipation
- Induces healthy bowel movements
- Keeps the gut satiated for long, thereby

suppressing appetite and promoting healthy weight loss

In this chapter, we speak about the many different food sources of prebiotics and how they work to keep our gut orderly despite the many different varieties of infection our gut is subjected to regularly.

The foods rich in prebiotics are broadly classified into 5 categories: cereal grains, vegetables, fruits, legumes, and nuts and seeds. Prebiotics exist in almost all fruits and vegetables as well as a variety of other foods as well. These are an exclusive class of nutrients that work to stimulate the good bacteria in the gut.

Let's dissect each of these categories and delve into more details regarding their prebiotic and other nutritional content. [41, 42]

1. CEREAL GRAINS

- **Oats:**

If there's an all-in-one choice for vegans, it has to be oats. This underrated cereal comes with umpteen dietary benefits, including antioxidative and anti-inflammatory properties, that are just hard to ignore.

The prebiotic fiber content in oats is 15.4 g per 100 g, which is quite exceptional.

Oats are the perfect breakfast choice, even for babies and diabetic people. It is rich in protein, healthy carbs, and antioxidants while being completely devoid of sugar. Just include a handful of oat grains in your regular recipes for porridges, smoothies, or soups, and you'll witness a noticeable difference in your gut health within a couple of weeks.

- **Bran:**

A grain of wheat is made up of three distinct layers: the bran, endosperm, and germ. The bran is the tough, outermost layer, while the germ is the innermost one, with the endosperm sandwiched between them.

Usually, when the wheat grains are milled to form flour, the bran is whisked away. However, the bran is jam-packed with nutritional fiber that is best suited for the gut. It is devoid of sugar, promotes healthy bowel movement, and reduces cholesterol in the long run.

Health experts always recommend consuming whole grains with their bran intact. Some types of bread are also baked with flour from whole grain cereals to retain the nutty flavor from wheat bran.

- **Barley:**

Barley is full of fiber, protein, carbs, and a healthy mix of vitamins and minerals. Prebiotic fiber is abundantly present in barley along with its immune-boosting and antioxidative properties.

Some studies also show how barley aids in weight loss and cholesterol reduction. It is even proven to improve digestion and regulate blood sugar levels. These benefits of barley aid in keeping your gut in shape and promote smooth bowel movements.

2. VEGETABLES

- **Chicory**

Chicory is a root fiber of a plant that belongs to the dandelion family. Inulin is an excellent prebiotic fiber found in abundance in chicory. The chicory root fiber has antioxidant properties and can alleviate constipation.

It is also used to prepare decoctions, as an alternative to coffee, as a food additive, and as a dietary supplement, especially to alleviate constipation or weak gut health. The exceptional taste of chicory makes it quite a sought-after additive in packaged foods.

Although chicory is an excellent source of prebiotic fiber, it may sometimes cause gas and bloating when consumed in excess. Pregnant and lactating women are also advised to avoid chicory for the same reasons.

- **Jerusalem artichokes**

This is a root tuber plant, pink and brown in color, that is native to Central America. Artichokes are high in prebiotic content and low in carbs as well. In other words, excess consumption of artichokes will only benefit your gut health and won't translate into unhealthy weight gain.

On average, this vegetable contains about 1.6 g of dietary fiber per 100 g of artichokes. Since artichokes are low in carbs, they also have a low glycemic index which regulates blood sugar levels too. It is your best bet to help improve the state of the good bacteria in your gut in the long run.

It has an abundance of antioxidative and anti-inflammatory properties. Artichokes can be consumed in a variety of ways and find a place in the diets of many cultures across the world.

- **Garlic**

One of the most commonly available foods in households and a significant part of every home remedy, garlic is just the right food for gut health. It is one of the best sources of prebiotics that promote the growth of beneficial gut bacteria and prevents harmful bacteria from multiplying.

The rich flavor of garlic makes its way into almost all types of foods, either after a slight sauté or giving it a burned flavor. Garlic instantly brings out the taste of breads, soups, sandwiches, and rice, along with improving it in nutritive content.

- **Onions, shallots, and spring onions**

Onions and shallots are abundantly present in all common dishes, especially in Asian cuisines. Spring onions also make for a good garnishing agent in soups, porridges, and rice dishes for that extra oomph in flavor.

These three belong to the same family of vegetables responsible for aiding in the digestion and metabolism of food and boosting beneficial gut health. They also boast immense antioxidative and anti-inflammatory properties.

- **Leeks**

Leeks are vegetables belonging to the onion family. They look like large green onions but have a creamier texture and a mild sweet flavor when cooked. The fiber content of leeks is about 1.8 g per 100 g and is quite an impressive amount.

Its anti-inflammatory properties help boost gut health and heart health while its rich prebiotic fiber content smooths digestion and metabolism to a large extent. Not only are leeks nutritious, but also quite easy to add to one's diet as well.

They can be eaten raw or sautéed and made part of veg salads. They even work well as a garnish or a side dish. Make sure to add a bit of leeks into your diet wherever you can to gain that healthy touch of nourishment.

- **Savoy cabbage**

Savoy cabbage makes for plenty of interesting, healthy dishes with the perfect mix of vitamins, minerals, and prebiotic fiber. It is the best dietary alternative for gut health as compared to most other options in the vegan category.

In addition to benefiting gut health, cabbage is perfect for cardiovascular health as well. The nutrition from cabbage helps regulate blood pressure, heart rate, and cholesterol levels. Cabbage is quite an easy addition to foods since it can be eaten as salads or in dishes, raw or cooked, or even simply tossed and seasoned minimally.

Vitamins like K, B, and C, and minerals like potassium combined with prebiotic fiber make it an exceptional choice for good gut health. Raw savoy cabbage makes a healthy addition to salads since it contains 3.1 g of fiber per 100 g of cabbage.

3. FRUITS

- **Bananas**

The main characteristic that makes bananas stand apart from other fruits is their perfect blend to satiate your hunger *and* thirst. Bananas are 75% water, meaning your gut will thank you for eating them! Water and fiber are crucial to keep your gut system in place and have it functioning smoothly.

Bananas are made up of 2.6 g of fiber per 100 g of fruit. While this is not the best ratio, it is certainly good for the gut, given bananas' amount of hydration.

Bananas are best consumed for breakfast as smoothies or as toppings on your cereal. They help ease constipation issues and reduce bloating. Other health benefits of bananas include regulating blood sugar levels, supporting heart health, and keeping you satiated for long.

- **Custard apples**

The antioxidative properties of custard apple are hard to ignore. The smooth texture and the sweetness of the fruit make it instantly enjoyable to consume directly or in desserts and milkshakes.

The heart and brain benefit primarily from antioxidants in general. Custard apples also aid in cholesterol reduction and regulation of glucose in the blood. As far as gut health is concerned, this fruit contains an abundance of prebiotic fiber that feeds the good bacteria in the gut, contributing to a robust gut microbiome over time.

- **Watermelon**

The watermelon boasts of being 92% water! It is the best fruit for the perfect mix of prebiotic fiber and hydration from water. Both these classes of nutrients are essential to keep the gut working at its finest.

The essential properties of watermelon also lower oxidative stress, curb inflammation, and help promote heart health. It aids in digestion too. The good effects of watermelon reflect in the form of glossy hair and supple skin.

- **Grapefruit**

It is imperative to include at least one citrus fruit in our diet each day: sweet lime, tangerine, or grapefruit. Grapefruit is rich in fiber, vitamins A and C, and substantially low in carbs. The nutrients derived from grapefruit strengthen immunity and play a significant role in regulating appetite levels.

4. LEGUMES

- **Chickpeas**

Plant-based fiber and protein is the best source of nutrition for the gut. Chickpeas, therefore, are perfect in this regard. They are packed with nutritional content, prebiotic fiber, and protein. 12.2 g of fiber per 100 g of chickpeas is quite a good deal for the gut.

Chickpeas are also quite versatile in terms of flavor and texture. There are a variety of ways you can cook them and create multiple dishes with the same nutritional value without getting bored of eating the same dish over and over again.

Since chickpeas are quite satiating, they help keep your appetite under control. Regulating blood sugar levels, improving digestion and metabolism, and strengthening immunity against chronic disorders are some of the many health benefits of chickpeas.

- **Lentils**

Lentils are one of the most underrated foods that provide ample nutrition with satiating qualities. They're filling, easy to digest, and full of protein, vitamins, and minerals. These inexpensive and underrated legumes are a staple food in the eastern world, although, currently, Canada is the leading producer of lentils worldwide.

Lentils contain about 10.8 g fiber per 100 g. They stimulate the good bacteria in the gut leading to smooth digestion and faster metabolism. Since they're a rich source of protein, they're often used in protein-rich diets to build muscle mass.

- **Red kidney beans, baked beans, and soybeans**

Baked beans are a popular breakfast food in the western world due to their rich protein and fiber content. The prebiotic fiber and the healthy blend of nutrition present in beans make it the perfect choice for building a good gut microbiome.

These are abundantly available, satiating, and inexpensive. Beans help boost gut health and immunity, address obesity, irregular blood sugar levels, and reduce blood pressure when consumed regularly.

Soybeans are a popular food across global cultures mainly used for fermentation with salt and bacteria. Many Korean and Chinese dishes stem from fermented soybeans, which are an excellent source of probiotics as well.

5. NUTS AND SEEDS

- **Almonds**

Almonds are an abundance of antioxidants, prebiotic fiber (12.5 g per 100 g), and a whole lot of other essential nutrients. Many studies have proven the benefits of almonds on brain and heart health.

They assist in regulating blood sugar and largely aid gut health by improving the quality of the gut microbiome. Almonds work like magic in keeping you satiated, which, in turn, prevents overeating due to hunger.

In addition to these nutritional benefits, almonds are rich in flavor and texture. They prove to be amazing add-ons for desserts, ice cream, cakes, and a wide range of hot and cold dishes.

- **Pistachio nuts**

Pistachios are such a widely popular dry fruit, largely present in every home. They contain abundant vegetable protein, antioxidants, prebiotic fiber, dietary fiber, vitamins, and minerals.

Since pistachios are low in calories and high in protein content, they prove to be wonderful for healthy and safe weight loss. The nutrition from pistachios stimulates good gut bacteria and aids in smooth bowel movements along with promoting blood vessel health.

- **Flaxseeds**

If you're looking for an inexpensive yet great source of healthy prebiotic fiber, phenolic acids, and antioxidants, then your search ends with flaxseeds. They are not just incredible for your gut microbiome but also regulate gut health, ease bowel movements, and control blood sugar levels.

In addition to this, flaxseeds impart an excellent flavor to various dishes like smoothies, desserts, and porridges. They're a versatile seed that can bring up the flavor of any dish by several notches.

QUICK RECAP

Prebiotic fiber is one of the essential classes of nutrients required by the gut and, hence, the human body. While it is not a direct energy source like carbs and fats, it plays a major role in stimulating gut bacteria to perform better.

The gut bacteria rely upon the prebiotics to increase it in quality and the probiotics to add to the family of the microbiota quantitatively. Many foods are not just rich in prebiotics but also in other categories of nutrition as well.

If you're actively looking to improve your gut health, choose the right kinds of food, supplement your diet with these edibles, and keep a close tab on how your body responds. You can then regulate your diet accordingly.

6

THE POWER OF PROBIOTICS

The gut microbiome is a complex family consisting of various flora and fauna that decides the state of the gut. The gut bacteria are a small portion of the larger picture that includes everything existing in the gut microbiome. [47]

Gut micro-organisms consist of bacteria, viruses, protozoa, fungi, and yeasts. These make up trillions of microbes that are responsible for gut health. The microbial cells are unique to every individual, including siblings and twins.

Age, lifestyle, mode of birth, early childhood upbringing, and dietary habits all play significant roles in determining the strength of the gut microbiota. Probiotics exist in the urinary tract, lungs, vagina, skin, mouth, and large quantities in the gut.

A microbe is classified as probiotic if they…

… have an independent bodily function
… can survive inside the gut
… benefit gut health
… can be safely consumed orally.

What Are Probiotics, and How Do They Work?

Probiotics, as the name suggests, is a class of live bacteria and yeasts. These bacteria already live in the gut but also need to be supplemented through the diet. However, these bacteria are suitable for the gut. The gut microbiota contains a mix of both types of bacteria: good and bad. [50]

These two types of bacteria are constantly at war with one another. The side that we strengthen is the side that wins. The good, healthy bacteria in our gut needs to be backed by probiotics. A healthy dose of probiotics is imperative in strengthening the immune system, controlling inflammation, and breaking down complex matter in the diet.

They help digest and absorb the dietary matter, in addition to assimilating the nutrients into the bloodstream.

Probiotics also reduce the negative effects of antibiotics, lower pH levels, relieve diarrhea, and ease constipation.

The digestive system needs a constant supply of probiotics to aid in the metabolism and assimilation of food and keep the gut environment healthy and sound. The good news is that we don't need to consume probiotic supplements to meet this requirement. A diet full of fiber and healthy probiotics is sufficient to maintain a fit and fine gut. [48]

WHAT ARE THE DIFFERENT STRAINS OF PROBIOTICS?

The most common types of helpful bacterial strains include ***Lactobacillus*** and ***Bifidobacterium***. These are abundantly available in stores and are also present in probiotic supplements. Another common example of probiotic includes ***Saccharomyces boulardii.***

Yogurt, one of the most sought-after foods for probiotics, contains ***Streptococcus thermophillus*** and ***Lactobacillus bulgaricus*** in abundance. All these bacteria enter our gut through the food we eat, live inside our systems, multiply and grow, and help boost the overall gut health. They aid in digestion, metabolism, assimilation, and strengthening the immunity of your system.

CONSUMING PROBIOTICS AS PER YOUR NEED

Probiotics, generally, are just right for your gut health. One needs to consume a healthy mix of all types of probiotics to benefit your gut in every way. However, if one is dealing with a particular type of gut disorder like Crohn's disease or leaky gut, they should increase their probiotic intake for a faster and smoother recovery.

An imbalance in the gut microbiota calls for an excess intake of healthy probiotics to undo the damage. These negative effects usually arise due to a heavy intake of junk food, antibiotic medications which kill both good and bad microbiota, inflammation, emotional and physical stress, and immune dysfunction. [51]

A general rule of thumb when getting started on probiotics is to go for dietary sources and not supplements. Dietary sources like yogurt, kefir, kimchi, and different types of cheeses are some excellent sources of probiotics. If you're looking to boost your gut health, increase the intake of these foods in your diet.

Probiotics can cause bloating and gas at first. Taking probiotic supplements initially often causes discomfort in the gut. But it only gets better and more beneficial with time.

While probiotics are generally regarded as safe, some conditions make consuming heavy doses of probiotics difficult. Inflammation, compromised immunity, or a weak gut may stand in the way of experiencing the benefits of probiotic supplements. [53]

The best way is to start with a generic probiotic strain and build your way up from there. See if an overall beneficial, common strain of probiotic works for your gut. If not, you can then switch to another strain until you find one that gives you the best results.

Here are some of the most popular and beneficial foods that are rich sources of probiotics. Make it a point to include one or two of these items in your daily diet for a regular, steady intake of healthy probiotics. [55, 56]

1. Yogurt:

The first food that comes to mind when we speak of probiotics is yogurt. Yogurt is the perfect food to ease a disrupted gut. It works well to relax the insides of the GIT, especially in cases of constipation, nausea, diarrhea, or vomiting.

Not only is yogurt full of probiotics and good bacteria, but it is also a milk product. In other words, it is rich in calcium, vitamin B12, and potassium—the nutrients from yogurt help to absorb and balance out the amount of other minerals within our system.

Yogurt should be a compulsory food for the young and old alike to keep the gut in shape and help strengthen the gut microbiome in the long run. Iodine, a mineral required in minute quantities to maintain healthy thyroid function, is abundantly present in yogurt.

A healthy dose of iodine daily through the diet is just what you need to keep your metabolism sailing without any hiccups. The benefits of yogurt are plenty-fold and, hence, make it a compulsory addition to your meals at least once a day to maintain a happy gut.

2. Kefir:

A rich, fermented drink made by adding kefir grains to cow or goat milk, kefir rightly finds itself a due spot on this list. Unlike naturally occurring cereal grains, kefir grains are made from lactic acid derivatives and have a cauliflower-like appearance.

It is an abundant source of calcium since it is a milk derivative. Studies have shown that kefir is an underrated food for great gut health, full of probiotics, and richer in antibacterial properties than its popular counterpart, yogurt.

An oversensitive immune system can pave the way for opportunistic infections like allergies and asthma. Kefir backs up your immunity and tackles various food sensitivities so that your gut becomes strong enough to digest and metabolize most food substances.

Due to its amazing health benefits, kefir is quite a sought-after food when it comes to dealing with osteoporosis or bone health. Kefir is pretty easy to make and quite rich in beneficial properties for men, women, young, and old alike.

3. Sauerkraut:

This side dish originally hails from China, but the name is derived from Germany. Sauerkraut is a type of fermented cabbage that has been shredded, aged, and treated with lactic acid bacteria. Its nutritional benefits largely surpass those of fresh cabbage.

Sauerkraut is highly popular in European countries. Due to its sour, salty flavor, people use it as a side dish or topping to add an extra oomph to their meals. Since it is fermented, it can be stored in an air-tight container for months on end.

It is rich in probiotic properties and contains fiber and vitamins B, C, and K. Minerals like sodium, iron, and manganese are abundantly present in sauerkraut, making it the perfect food to improve your gut health naturally and safely.

4. Tempeh:

Tempeh is a traditional Indonesian dish made with fermented soybeans. It can be baked or sautéed or seasoned with various flavors depending on one's preference. The soybeans are pressed into a firm cake-like structure post-fermentation and used as a rich source of protein. There are many ways of customizing this dish.

Because of its rich protein content, tempeh is widely used globally as a vegetarian substitute for meat and meat products. Its nutty flavor and grainy texture add to its charm and make it the perfect staple dish for good gut health.

The abundance of protein, fiber, probiotics, and other nutrients in tempeh can be attributed to its soybean content and fermentation process. It is perfect for keeping your gut environment healthy and sound and enabling the gut microbiome to perform increasingly well over time.

Soybeans typically contain high amounts of phytic acid that can stand in the way of the smooth absorption of vitamins and minerals. However, the fermentation process decreases the phytic content, enabling the gut to absorb all the nutrients in tempeh without any hiccups.

5. Kimchi:

Kimchi hails from the traditional concept of storing and preserving vegetables for a long time, since cultivation wasn't always possible under harsh climatic conditions. A fermented, spicy Korean dish that consists of a variety of vegetables fermented and stored in salt and vinegar.

People choose to add various seasonings and a mix of other add-ins as well, like garlic, red chili pepper flakes, or ginger to improve the flavor and nutritional value of this dish. Cabbage is the main ingredient, but kimchi can also contain other veggies like radish, carrot, cucumber, and beetroot.

Kimchi contains lactic acid bacteria called Lactobacillus, which are perfect for improving gut health and digestion. Besides containing probiotics, kimchi is quite nutrient-dense as well. It has plenty of antioxidative and anti-inflammatory properties that slow down aging and strengthen the immune system respectively.

6. Miso:

Miso is a thick paste made from fermenting soybeans with salt and a fungus called koji and seasoned with a variety of flavors. While soybeans are the original base ingredient in the making of miso, some people use other types of beans or peas for a healthy change in flavor or texture.

Miso is an excellent dish for a rich intake of probiotics regularly. Miso is often mixed with soybeans and other ingredients like barley, rice, and rye to improve its nutritional content. In addition to that, it has vitamins, minerals, and plant fibers abundantly present in it, thereby imparting better nutritive abilities.

A blend of fiber and probiotics is just what the gut needs to keep performing optimally. And miso gives you that perfect combination in the right quantity. It improves digestion, promotes a faster metabolism, and strengthens overall immunity in the body.

7. Kombucha:

Kombucha is a type of fermented black or green tea drink which dates back centuries. It is rich in probiotics and has excellent anti-inflammatory and antioxidative properties. Interestingly, kombucha is one of the most sought-after beverages in many parts of the world, especially in Asia.

The fermentation process of kombucha occurs due to a friendly colony of bacteria and yeast. It contains the beneficial effects of both green/black tea and the probiotic content.

The nutritional content in kombucha helps regulate heart rate, control blood sugar levels, ease constipation and bowel movements, and promote good gut health over time.

8. Pickles:

Pickles are famous across the world for their tangy and refreshing flavor. These are marinated cucumbers that have been soaked in a solution of salt and water. These pieces of cucumbers ferment within this solution, undergo a chemical alteration within their own lactic-acid-producing bacteria, and turn sour in the process. This sour taste gives them their unique flavor.

The bacteria make their way into the pickles, making them an excellent alternative for promoting good gut health. Pickles are full of minerals, good probiotic bacteria, vitamin K, and naturally, low in calories and unhealthy carbs.

Vitamin K is essential to induce blood clotting in case of injuries to prevent extreme blood loss. A major drawback here is that pickles are high in sodium content due to the excess amount of salt added for fermentation and preservation.

9. Traditional Buttermilk:

Buttermilk, the leftover milk after butter is churned, is known as buttermilk. This traditional drink is also known as "Grandma's probiotic" and is exceptionally rich in good bacteria perfect for gut health. This drink is easier on the gut since it is simpler to digest, may strengthen bones, and is also known to regulate cholesterol levels.

Nowadays, buttermilk is available in many different varieties that contain added bacterial cultures. This modern type of buttermilk is richer in texture and flavor and is often used to make cakes, cookies, and other baked items.

The traditional version of buttermilk is the best for your gut health. A fresh glass of this drink instantly lifts your mood, replenishes your energy levels, and soothes your gut. Just like yogurt and kefir impart antibacterial and cooling properties in the gut, so does traditionally made buttermilk sans the unrequired additives.

10. Natto:

Just like tempeh, natto is also a fermented soybean dish. It is pretty rich in probiotic bacterial content. It has a slimy, stringy texture which is disliked by many. However, natto has an acquired taste. Its nutty flavor and sticky texture later grow on the palate.

Natto is pretty common in Japan and is a staple in the Japanese diet. It is extremely rich in other nutrients as well like protein, vitamin K2, and calcium. Japanese people usually season natto with mustard and soy sauce and serve it with cooked rice for breakfast.

A blend of probiotics coupled with the other nutrients from natto is perfect for gut health. It also promotes bone and cardiovascular health.

11. Some types of cheeses:

Milk and milk products are rich in calcium, and fermented milk products are great sources of healthy bacteria for the gut. Although all types of cheese are fermented, not all cheeses contain probiotics. The best way to find out if a type of cheese is best for you is to study the food labels on it.

Cottage cheese, cheddar cheese, Gouda, mozzarella, Parmesan, and Swiss are some varieties of cheese rich in probiotics. When cheeses age, some strains of bacteria survive the aging process, thereby increasing the bacterial levels.

In addition to probiotics, cheese is also an amazing source of vitamins like B12 and minerals like calcium, phosphorous, and selenium.

However, one must keep tabs on their consumption of cheese to avoid excess intake of fat. A moderate amount of cheese in the diet may also reduce the risk of heart disease and osteoporosis.

QUICK RECAP

Probiotics are a class of good bacteria that exist in the gut and need to be supplemented through the diet to maintain a healthy state of the gut environment.

They're responsible for strengthening the good bacteria in the gut, building immunity, and fending off any foreign infections at the earliest.

Foods rich in probiotics exist in all cultures worldwide, and most of them are fermented with different types of bacteria. This fermentation process makes it possible to store these foods without fear of them going bad.

In addition to that, it increases the probiotic content in these foods, thereby adding to the overall nutritional value. Consuming a mix of foods rich in probiotics, fiber, vitamins, and minerals is just what your gut needs to stay robust and keep performing optimally over time.

7

WORST FOODS FOR YOUR GUT

The core aspect of good health is mainly made up of a good diet, followed by strict exercise routines and, lastly, healthy lifestyle habits. We are well aware of the goodness of various foods and how they work to raise our gut health by several levels.

However, in the same category, a vast majority of us forget to exclude certain foods that negate the health benefits of our good diets. Just like it is essential to include healthy foods in our diet for the maintenance of the gut, it is equally important to cut down on harmful substances that further degrade the quality of our gut system.

Good foods for gut health promote the quantitative and qualitative growth of the good bacteria in the gut, and excessively eating harmful foods contributes to the development of bad bacteria which is detrimental to gut health.

Individuals whose diet comprises a healthy blend of veg and non-veg foods, coupled with a supervised intake of dietary supplements, are at the best advantage as far as their gut health is concerned.

If your workout regime is in place, lifestyle habits are immaculate, and your diet contains a good mix of all essential nutrients, but you are still consuming foods that are harmful to the gut, it can take a heavy toll on your overall health.

It is not enough to exercise and change your lifestyle habits because the diet needs to be correct. All your efforts in the right direction will bear no fruit if not backed by the proper dietary habits, including cutting down on foods detrimental to gut health.

Several other factors come into play when deciding how a food item performs in the gut. Sometimes, due to certain allergies or sensitivities, an individual may suffer from gastrointestinal issues due to an otherwise gut-friendly edible. [57, 58, 59, 60]

All foods that work like slow poison for the gut can are grouped into 4 broad categories. These help us differentiate between the various types of food and how they affect the gut.

- **Animal protein:**

Animal protein is one of the most crucial sources of protein for the human body. In fact, vegans need to go that extra mile to fill their void of protein that is abundantly available in the meal choices for non-vegetarian eaters.

Eggs, dairy, lean meat, seafood, and red meat are rich in protein and provide a perfect culmination of essential vitamins and minerals, like choline, for the smooth upkeep of our system.

The only drawback here is that humans should not consume animal protein in excess. A heavy intake of non-veg foods each day only bulks up the quantity of animal protein that we consume regularly. This, in turn, leads to a steady decline in the performance of the gut.

The gut and gut microbiome work harder to digest animal protein than they need to for other nutrients or protein from vegan sources. Therefore, people who constantly consume diets that are very high in animal protein may suffer some harmful changes in their gut microbiome.

It is best to consume animal protein every other day or every 3 days to allow your gut time to "rest." This habit ensures that the gut stays functioning at its best.

Since the gut microbiome is heavily employed when it needs to digest animal protein, the inner lining of the intestines undergoes extra "duties" as well. Therefore, a constant supply of animal protein within the gut will take a serious toll on health.

The erosion and inflammation of the gut walls upon heavy intake of animal protein is a common phenomenon. It can culminate in inflammatory bowel disorder, or further plummet into other unwanted conditions like a leaky gut.

Recent research on the gut diversity of two sets of children shed light on a whole new perspective. This study was initiated to study the gut bacteria of some children from Italy and another group of children from a rural area in Burkina Faso in Africa.

The former set of subjects had a diet comprising meat and animal products, while the latter consumed a diet high in plant fiber and pea protein. The rural children showed a more diverse set of gut microbiomes than the urban children.

This could also be because the urban diet is a little less contaminated than the rest of the country. This lack of exposure to all types of bacteria results in a less diverse gut microbiome that can withstand serious foreign infections.

The gut microbiota of the urban children from Italy was primarily associated with inflammation and other disorders, while the African children sported a more robust gut family devoid of probable diseases.

- **Fried foods:**

A general notion among the common public is that oil is unhealthy. While that is partially true, there is some more truth to add to that. Oils, or rather fats, predominantly occur in three forms: saturated, unsaturated, and trans fats.

Without delving into the core details of each of these types, let's say that unsaturated fats are the good fats for your body while saturated and trans fats only come with adverse effects. The oil used for frying food like is usually rich in saturated and trans fats.

Trans fats are abundantly present in packaged foods like chips, burgers, and donuts. They have a huge hand in leading your body to obesity and heart health issues.

The components of fried food irritate the gut walls' inner lining, thereby leading to diarrhea, gas, bloating, and stomach pains. The liver also suffers greatly when our diet is not aligned with the needs of the gut. The risk of liver disease increases by several notches when the diet is heavily influenced by fried food.

Therefore, doctors advise people with liver health issues to cut down on fried, packaged, and sugary foods as the first step to improving their diet and setting their eating habits right. Any malfunction in the liver can become a cause of gastrointestinal disorders, leaky gut, or other diseases of the gut.

Sugar and fried foods are hazardous to health but highly palatable. Fast food chains run on the flavor produced by sugar and fried foods, creating a mild addiction that causes people, especially children, to crave it more!

- **Sugar:**

One of the worst foods for the human body, highly detrimental to mental and physical health, is sugar. Refined or processed sugar promotes the number of antioxidants in our system that catalyze the overall body's aging and individual vital systems.

Naturally occurring sugars, like in fruits, are a form of carbohydrate and are, therefore, good for our body and mind. But refined sugar produces just the opposite effect.

Refined sugar is obtained by extracting natural sugar from sugar cane, sugar beets, or corn.

This processed, refined sugar, often known as table sugar, makes its way into our desserts, coffees, cookies, and other dishes. It is general knowledge that sugar is unhealthy for our vital systems, but very few know why it is so.

As we've understood so far, the root cause of all gut health disorders begins with inflammation. And sugar is one of the leading contributors to gut inflammation. It not only gets in the way of smooth digestion of the system but also actively harms gut diversity and dampens the function of the gut microbiome.

Excess sugar degrades the intestines' mucosal barrier, leading to dysbiosis and breakage in the intestinal walls. Dysbiosis, a reduction in gut microbial diversity, coupled with a compromised permeability of the intestinal walls, is the perfect recipe for a leaky gut.

Not only does excess sugar get in the way of good gut health, but it also has knock-on effects for other vital systems. It contributes to excess blood sugar, promotes cardiovascular disorders, induces weight gain, and can permanently alter the function of gut bacteria for the worse.

Sugar, along with empty calories and processed foods, plays a huge role in pushing one toward obesity in the long run. Once obesity sets in, the gut microbiome is altered entirely and permanently. The microbial life in the gut is heavily compromised and produces a negative domino effect on the functioning of the rest of the body as well.

- **Processed foods:**

Processed foods are an obvious cause. They are full of trans fats, sugar, and other harmful components that hinder the gut's smooth functioning. While a diet that is heavily reliant on processed meals instead of cooked food doesn't produce adverse effects directly, it does contribute to GI disorders in a big way.

We live in a world of fast and cheap food wherein health takes a back seat behind all other priorities. The urban lifestyle is super-fast-paced and hectic. Constantly consuming processed foods leads to toxic buildup in your system that takes a series of medications and lifestyle changes to undo.

Processed foods consist of all edible items that are not naturally occurring but consumed mainly in the name of food. Packaged food items like instant noodles, chips, fries, donuts, breakfast cereals, bread, cookies, desserts, savory snacks, and all types of ready-to-eat meals fall under the category of processed foods.

Such food items are exceptionally high in sugar, calories, and trans fats, in addition to being very low in fiber content. This combination of nutrients is enough to put your gut health in bad shape with only a few days of being on a processed foods diet.

This type of diet, with prolonged consumption, can raise the levels of LDL cholesterol in your system. LDL, or bad cholesterol, contributes to obesity and cardiovascular disorders.

SUMMING IT UP

Diet is everything. It can make or break a person's body. Regardless of how much one exercises and makes necessary lifestyle changes, it will be of little importance if not backed by a good diet. [64]

Being on a good diet is synonymous with eating foods that are good for the gut and body. But that's not all. A significant portion of a good diet includes cutting down on food that is hazardous to the gut and, hence, to the body's overall health.

When your goal is to lose weight safely and gain muscle mass, the first step is to cut down on sugar and fried and processed foods. The next step is to increase the intake of protein, fiber, and probiotics—all foods that pave the way to a healthy gut. [65, 66]

As mentioned in the previous chapters, the body's vital systems are interconnected. The functions are interdependent and are influenced by each other's smooth or disrupted functioning.

Hence, one's diet needs to be of top-notch quality to ensure a diverse gut microbiome that will translate into a strong immunity and an overall healthy body and mind.

QUICK RECAP

Just like some foods boost gut health, some foods bring it down too. Our responsibility toward our body is to recognize these foods, differentiate between them, and increase or decrease them in our diet based on the effects they bring.

Other factors like food sensitivities, allergies, age, overall diet patterns, habits developed in early childhood, and other lifestyle changes also govern how a food item will perform in the gut. However, some categories of food are hazardous for all, regardless of all other secondary factors.

Fried foods, packaged foods, sugar, processed meals, junk food, and excess animal protein are major red flags that will create havoc in the gut with disruptive qualities.

They cause inflammation, reduction in diversity, and compromise the permeability of the gut walls. These effects are detrimental by themselves and could also lead to further damage in and around the gut, thereby hampering the function of the rest of the systems as well.

8

LET'S TALK VITAMINS AND SUPPLEMENTS

Gut health is reliant on multiple factors in addition to diet and lifestyle. Often, our diet falls short of providing us with adequate nutrients. This can happen due to our dietary choices, dislike for certain foods, allergies, or sensitivities.

Cultural differences or malabsorption in the gut also prevent one from consuming certain foods that could otherwise add to the overall nutrient content in the diet. Owing to these factors, sometimes people suffer from deficiencies of essential minerals and vitamins in the diet. [67]

When this happens, it becomes crucial to consume dietary supplements to meet this increasing demand of the body. Even if there is no deficiency, it is always a good idea to consume dietary supplements to ensure an adequate and steady supply of essential nutrients for smooth gut function and overall wellness of the body. [68, 69]

NOTE: *Always consume FDA-approved dietary supplements under the strict guidance of your health professional. Age, lifestyle, medications, and medical history must all be considered before choosing the composition of your vitamin and mineral supplements.* [70, 71]

1. VITAMINS

The body needs two types of vitamins to function optimally: water-soluble and fat-soluble. The former type of vitamins (B and C) is easily absorbed by the digestive system, is readily photo-oxidized if left outside for long, and cannot be stored in the body when consumed in excess.

Fat-soluble vitamins (A, D, E, and K) can only be absorbed by the fat reserves in our system. When consumed in excess, these vitamins are not simply excreted but are stored within the body. A buildup of fat-soluble vitamins can lead to disorders within the system.

Vitamin B:

This is a class of vitamins essential to the body to maintain good gut health. Our body needs vitamin B to create red blood cells and impart energy to the gut to keep going. Primarily speaking, vitamin B12 is responsible for boosting gut health in a huge way.

Deficiency of vitamin B12 can lead to issues like diarrhea, cramping in the stomach, nausea, and poor gut health. The gut needs iron to function optimally, and iron needs B12 to get absorbed properly into the gut.

A healthy intake of B vitamins ensures that your gut bacteria thrive in a stable, steady environment. They back up your gut health like no other dietary supplement and must make their way into your meals to complement a healthy, balanced diet.

Vitamin C:

Vitamin C is a water-soluble vitamin and is richly present in citrus fruits like oranges, sweet limes, pomegranates, lemon, and grapefruit. It is an excellent antioxidant that slows down the effects of aging along with boosting immunity as well.

It is imperative to consume healthy amounts of vitamin C in our diet to ensure healthy gums and teeth. Poor dental health and bleeding gums are the first signs of a deficiency of vitamin C in the body. Consume your citrus fruits daily for a healthy intake of vitamin C in your diet.

However, it is best to eat your fruits and not just rely on fruit juices since water-soluble vitamins are readily photo-oxidized. While vitamin C is abundantly available in all our daily food items, taking dietary supplements helps boost immunity and reduce the effects of aging on our bodies.

Vitamin D:

Our skin receptors synthesize vitamin D within the body when exposed to the early morning rays of the sun. Consuming vitamin D in healthy quantities has been linked to the prevention of colon cancer as per a study conducted in 2015.

Vitamin D and calcium go hand in hand. The absence of one also leads to the deficiency of another. Vitamin D is crucial to help the body absorb calcium from food. Without vitamin D, our body cannot absorb calcium which leads to calcium deficiency as well.

A deficiency of vitamin D usually occurs when an individual spends too much time indoors and doesn't step out into the sun often. Since we spend most of our time indoors, it is best to include vitamin D supplements in our diet to ensure a steady supply of essential nutrients in our system.

2. MINERALS

Our body needs minerals in minute quantities, but they are crucial for good health nevertheless. These minerals play varying roles in our body like regulating blood sugar levels, maintaining electrolyte balance, and enhancing gut function.

A balanced diet including fruits, vegetables, and pulses is enough to ensure a healthy intake of minerals like calcium, potassium, and iron.

Selenium:

The major function of selenium is boosting gut health. Selenium protects the inner lining of the gut and enhances your gut's response to inflammation.

An inflamed gut is the root cause of many health issues in the body, and they're better nipped in the bud itself. A dearth of selenium in the diet creates a heightened stress response and increases inflammatory levels in the body.

Other benefits of selenium include boosting immune health, improving thyroid function, reducing symptoms of asthma, and it works as a potent antioxidant.

Magnesium:

Magnesium is one of the most widely present minerals in almost all our food items. It is practically impossible to fall short of magnesium in the diet if you are consuming a variety of foods from all categories. The key role of magnesium is to relax your muscles, balance your blood sugar levels, cope with stress, and minimize inflammation within your gut.

Magnesium supplements only ensure that these functions take place optimally in addition to improving gut health in the long run. Most magnesium supplements contain magnesium citrate, which has three times the absorption rate compared to other types of magnesium supplements.

Iron:

Iron is a crucial component in the blood vessels. The red blood cells, RBCs, need iron in minute amounts to function optimally. In addition to that, iron is known for boosting immunity, enhancing gut health, improving muscle endurance, and increasing hemoglobin production as well.

The good bacteria in the gut use iron from the diet to function better. In fact, a National Center for Biotechnology study found that iron supplementation increased an anti-inflammatory bacterial metabolite and enhanced the number of gut bacteria.

While iron is widely present in leafy greens, dietary supplementation works best to ensure a healthy, adequate, and steady supply of the same in our diet.

Zinc:

Zinc plays a major role in regulating blood sugar levels, improving cardiovascular health, and slows down macular degeneration over time. With regard to gut health, zinc works best for boosting the production of digestive enzymes.

This, in turn, prevents leaky gut syndrome and catalyzes weight loss in the long run. For best results, zinc supplements should only be consumed under the guidance of your health professional.

3. FATTY ACIDS

Omega-3:

Essential fatty acids, unlike non-essential fatty acids, cannot be synthesized within the body and need to be consumed in the diet. Omega-3 is an essential fatty acid that is responsible for reducing inflammation, controlling unhealthy cholesterol levels, improving cognitive health, and boosting cardiovascular conditions for better overall health of our body.

The antioxidative properties of omega-3s are crucial to reduce aging, promote skin health, stimulate hair growth, and decrease the other signs of aging as well. Studies have also shown that omega-3 fatty acids may contribute to increasing the good bacteria in the gut for a smooth digestive and metabolic function.

QUICK RECAP

Even the best dietary supplements for vitamins, minerals, fiber, and fatty acids are no match for the naturally available nutrients in the diet. Hence, try to consume as much essential nourishment from your diet as possible to bypass the possibilities of any side effects or allergic reactions.

Having said that, dietary supplementation is your best bet to help maintain the health of your body when one's diet fails to provide the same.

9

LEAKY GUT

The hollow organs of the gut, namely the esophagus, stomach, and intestines, have highly rigid walls to keep their contents limited to within the organ. The walls of these organs, especially the intestines, are ***permeable.***

In other words, these walls allow the passage of molecules through them. This permeability of the intestinal walls enables the enzymes from the liver and pancreas to enter the intestines and metabolize the digestive matter. [72]

Permeability also releases the absorbed nutritive substances from the intestine to enter the bloodstream and get assimilated to the different parts of the body.

UNDERSTANDING LEAKY GUT

The permeability of the intestinal walls is essential, without which the gut will not be able to perform at its optimum. However, sometimes this permeability increases more than required. The tight junctions of the gut walls become unable to monitor the passage of molecules from and within the gut. This condition is known as ***leaky gut***. [73, 74]

All the toxic and nitrogenous waste is collected and expelled through the anus eventually. Under ideal circumstances, the gut only releases the nourishing substances into the bloodstream and keeps the toxic waste within.

But when the gut walls lose their control, the toxins and undigested food particles slowly seep into the bloodstream and start affecting the nearby organs.

As a result, the damage to the gut walls leads to conditions like inflammation, autoimmune responses, weakened immunity, and severe allergic reactions.

These immediate effects eventually lead to visible health disorders like eczema, chronic fatigue, irritable bowel, food allergies, rheumatoid arthritis, and mental health conditions like depression and anxiety.

WHAT PHYSICAL CHANGES DOES THE GUT UNDERGO?

The intestines are a crucial part of the GIT and are closely involved in metabolism and assimilation. The final churning of the food matter also happens in the intestines, where the toxic waste is separated from the last bit of nutrition and discarded from the system forever. [75]

Therefore, these intestines are encased in an extensive lining that protects their contents from mixing into the outer atmosphere that lies beyond the gut walls. This lining is wrinkled on the surface but can easily cover 4000 sq. ft. of surface area if stretched out flat.

Under ideal circumstances, the intestinal covering is permeable but forms a tight barrier that controls the transfer from and within the gut. Any toxic waste or undigested food matter cannot escape into the blood-stream unless prompted by the intestinal walls.

However, in the case of a leaky gut, the gut lining suffers extensive physical damage. It develops cracks, lines, or holes that facilitate the entry of partially digested food particles, toxins, or bugs to percolate into the bloodstream, leading to a leaky gut.

The effects of a leaky gut worsen further because the bloodstream is not ready to receive such unexpected molecules from the gut. Therefore, a series of unwanted reactions take place, causing a visible decline in overall health.

Leaky gut may sound like a simple, manageable issue but it has graver impacts than it seems. The gut flora and fauna face severe implications due to this leakage. The gut microbiota diversity is highly compromised, thereby affecting immunity and causing improper absorption of nutrients from the food matter.

Current research shows, with such physical modifications in the intestinal walls and the gut, the microbiota can develop into several common chronic diseases if left untreated.

WHAT ARE THE SYMPTOMS OF LEAKY GUT?

Many symptoms of leaky gut coincide with poor gut health since a leaky gut is, after all, an unhealthy gut. Some of the significant red flags that point toward leaky gut include:

1. Digestive issues:

Digestive issues are the first major sign that your body uses to convey that there's something wrong with your gut. These digestive issues arise because the gut is unable to perform at its optimum level.

The gut walls continuously lose control over the transmission of molecules in a two-way passage, resulting in diarrhea, constipation, gas accumulation, and bloating.

Poor gut health is one of the core reasons why your gut health can be impaired. But if this condition persists and is accompanied by other symptoms, it only indicates a leaky gut.

2. Nutritional deficiencies:

A malfunctioning gut cannot absorb nutrients very well. It also happens when the undigested food molecules escape into the bloodstream through the gut walls without proper digestion and metabolism. That bit of nutrient gets lost forever and instead translates into inflammation and allergies in the nearby organs.

Nutritional deficiency, despite a well-balanced diet, is one of the significant signs of poor gut health. If other symptoms accompany it, it indicates that the problem is not just poor gut health but, in fact, a leaky gut.

3. Poor immune system:

A weak gut and a weak immune system go hand in hand. When the gut microbiota loses its diversity, it poses a direct threat to the immune system. A weak immune system is a perfect hub for opportunistic infections and allergies which further cause the body's overall strength to decline.

4. Mental health effects:

Headaches, brain fog, memory loss, depression, anxiety, or ADHD are becoming increasingly common as by-products of leaky gut syndrome. The molecules that leak into the bloodstream from the gut trigger inflammation near the liver and the pancreas.

This inflammation disturbs the secretion of serotonin in your system. ***Serotonin and dopamine***, also known as happy hormones, keep the happiness levels up in your mind and keep you feeling refreshed and content. When the serotonin levels in your system dip, it results in mental health issues like brain fog, anxiety, ADHD, ADD, and depression.

One of the major clinical treatments of mental health conditions includes administering serotonin and dopamine supplements to induce happiness and good feelings in the individual. A leaky gut is not the only cause of mental health issues but can be a leading factor.

5. Excessive fatigue:

Food sensitivities, allergies, digestive issues, bloating, and constipation are some of the most common signs of a leaky gut. If you're facing an unidentifiable reason for excessive fatigue coupled with digestive issues and mood swings, it is a condition of gut health being compromised over time.

6. Skin conditions:

Skin conditions like eczema, rosacea, spots, allergies, psoriasis, and rashes are some of the most indirect repercussions of a leaky gut. These skin conditions only arise when the body triggers inflammatory responses within the system.

This is a more visible and apparent response and doesn't manifest itself immediately. Only when the damaged intestinal barriers stay damaged for a prolonged period do they result in such visual skin conditions.

7. Unhealthy cravings:

Since the gut cannot absorb all nutrients from the food matter, the body starts becoming low in energy despite having a good diet. There occurs a deficiency of nutrients due to improper absorption and not because of an improper diet.

As a result, the body starts craving calories and other immediate energy sources like sugar and carbs. The need for those instant bursts of energy increases and compels you to consume sugary and oily food, mostly junk food like fries, burgers, and donuts.

8. Arthritis or joint pain:

Since the gut walls are less able to contain the matter within them, the toxic waste and undigested food particles seep into the bloodstream unwantedly. These molecules belong within the gut and not in the neighborhood interacting with vital organs.

But when that happens, it results in chronic inflammation that gets spread all through the system. As we already know, the root cause of arthritis is inflammation in the joints. Although arthritis is one of the many drawbacks of a leaky gut, it is not the only one. Similarly, a leaky gut is not the only cause of arthritis but can be a catalyzing factor as well.

9. Autoimmune diseases:

The immune system is always on the lookout for foreign particles around the gut to fend off. There are a host of other factors too that trigger immune responses in the body.

However, when the cells from the immune system come in contact with these toxins and undigested food particles that have oozed out of the intestinal walls, they fail to recognize them as part of the system. [74]

Furthermore, when these molecules trigger inflammatory responses in the vicinity of the gut, the immune system sets out to get rid of them, thereby destroying the cells and tissues from the vital organs in the bargain. This autoimmune response is one of the most common occurrences that points toward a leaky gut. [75]

WHAT CAUSES A LEAKY GUT?

Despite our best efforts, our gut sometimes doesn't exactly function at its optimal best. We may have the best diet with the best culmination of prebiotic and probiotic nutrition combined with a healthy dose of vitamins and supplements and live a healthy lifestyle.

But some unfortunate cases occur despite being on a well-balanced diet or having a healthy lifestyle. And a leaky gut is one such condition. Not that a good diet has no positive effects, but other factors come into play too. All aspects together have an impact on the gut.

These practical factors include environmental conditions, lifestyle habits, stress levels, medications, health disorders, age, and occupational hazards.

Although a poor diet can be a solid probable cause of a leaking gut, there can be other reasons. Our organs and systems sometimes malfunction due to improper overall care. Being on a good diet only addresses one aspect of looking after your body.

Of these, our diet and eating habits are the most crucial elements that decide the fate of our gut health. Any changes or imbalance in these factors can have a direct result on the condition of your gut. These are some of the determining factors and not the exact causes of what causes a leaky gut in the first place. [76]

Although the core reason for the permeability of the intestinal walls is yet unknown, research points out interesting evidence that can be considered as solid reasons for the same. Let's delve into some of these reasons and dissect this issue to understand what exactly causes a leaky gut.

Poor diet:

A poor diet lacking in nutrition combined with unhealthy, untimely eating habits is the number one cause of any issue related to the gut. As mentioned repeatedly, our food is directly received by the gut. Any goodness or harshness in the diet has direct consequences on our gut.

Hence, a poor diet devoid of prebiotic or probiotic nutrition, lacking in vitamins and minerals, or having a serious shortage of dietary fiber can cause gut health to be diminished.

Occasionally having an unhealthy meal full of sugar, carbs, or oily foods doesn't do much harm since the gut is strong enough to withstand it. But regularly consuming oily, fried, and sugary food without paying close attention to our daily nutrient intake culminates in severe gut disorders like, in this case, a leaky gut.

Dysbiosis:

Dysbiosis happens when the diversity of the gut microbiota starts declining at a heavy pace. As we know, our gut health directly relies on the diversity of our gut microbiota. The more diverse the bacteria are in the gut, the stronger the gut, and the better it is for the body.

However, if this diversity starts declining, the intestinal walls become less able to contain their contents within them as well as they could previously. [81]

You may wonder what causes this decline in the diversity of the gut microbiota? The reasons could be many. A poor diet, fluctuating eating habits, stress, medications, or other health disorders can reduce microbiome diversity in the gut.

Stressful lifestyle:

The gut-brain axis demonstrates the close connection between the working of the brain and the gut. Many tensed nerves in and around the intestinal walls can give way to its contents, thereby resulting in more permeability than necessary. Therefore, a stressed mind is fully capable of launching a stressful result on the gut as well.

While stress may not directly affect the intestinal walls, it can suppress one's appetite. A stressed mind results in a stressed gut which is not very prone to experiencing hunger as well. This may cause a drop in nutrition levels, thereby contributing to a leaky gut.

Toxin overload:

Our gut is rugged and powerful enough to withstand all sorts of infections and toxins. However, the gut might become weak if there's an overload of toxic intake. Generally speaking, the gut of an individual residing in an urban area leading a modern life is exposed to about 80,000 hazardous chemicals and toxins daily.

These can enter the body in a variety of ways, namely through junk food, contaminated food and water, polluted air, touching contaminated surfaces, exposed environmental conditions, and also due to occupational hazards.

The main channels through which toxins enter our body include pesticides, antibiotics, medicinal drugs, and contaminated edibles. This takes a heavy toll on the gut's health, thereby weakening it and causing leaky walls.

SUMMING IT UP

A leaky gut condition doesn't pop out of anywhere, nor does any improper care directly result in a leaky gut. A series of reactions occurs like a domino effect, one factor leading to another, which finally culminates in gut leakage.

For instance, a highly stressful lifestyle takes a toll on one's mental health, which suppresses the appetite, causes the diet to suffer, and prevents the gut from receiving good nutrition, which ultimately causes a leaky gut.

And it doesn't even stop there. A leaky gut has its own implications on other vital organs of the body and can cause improper absorption of nutrients, inflammation, and poor immunity.

HOW CAN ONE ADDRESS LEAKY GUT SYNDROME?

Before we get to the personal care habits to mend your leaky gut, there are some important aspects to consider:

- There is no substitute for medical care. Any malfunction within the system needs to be dealt with using proper medication under the guidance of a health professional.
- It is imperative to make healthy lifestyle changes in your regimen. Relying on medications and treatment alone is not enough.
- Medications, along with healthy lifestyle habits, work in tandem to improve your overall health. Both of these aspects are like two oars of the same boat.
- Give your mind and body some time to heal from the discomfort and after-effects of a leaky gut. Even if you start feeling better initially, it is best to complete your medical treatment and take precautions with plenty of rest to have a long-lasting recovery.

Getting to the heart of the subject, how exactly does one deal with a leaky gut?

The solutions are built along the same lines now that we know the probable causes of a leaky gut. The major steps include paying attention to one's diet, mental health, and fitness levels to address it.

- **Diet:**

Prebiotic fiber and probiotic foods work like magic to restore the lost strength and diversity of your gut. You cannot compromise on this step if you're looking to recover fast and well. Other nutrients include vitamins, minerals, fruits, dietary fiber, and plenty of hydration.

While on the topic, also reduce the intake of refined carbs. Refined carbs and sugar will surely satisfy your cravings but only worsen a leaky gut situation. Ensure all your food is thoroughly washed and not contaminated with insecticides or pesticides since they can damage gut health.

- **Medicinal drugs:**

One of the major possible reasons for a leaky gut is toxin overload due to medicinal drugs like antibiotics, analgesics, and NSAIDs. If contaminated with pesticides and insecticides, our food can also contribute to destroying the gut lining. Therefore, keep your drug usage to the bare minimum consuming only what is directly required to help your gut.

While antibiotics and NSAIDs, non-steroidal anti-inflammatory drugs, may seem like the right choice to counter pain and inflammation in the vital systems, they will only increase the toxin levels in your system. But you can always consume dietary supplements like vitamins and prebiotics.

- **Lifestyle changes:**

Stress, high alcohol intake, substance intake, and an unhealthy fitness regime are all major contributing factors to a leaky gut. These habits, when occurring simultaneously, can weaken your gut health over time, thereby compromising your immunity by a large margin.

When you're on the path to recovery, it is crucial to make necessary changes in your lifestyle as well. Reduce your stress levels, bring down your hectic work hours, incorporate a little physical activity or yoga in your daily schedule, and cut down any habitual alcohol or substance intake.

These improvements in lifestyle habits will culminate in a healthy gut and strong immunity which will erase all the negative impacts and symptoms that your body was dealing with.

QUICK RECAP

The gut walls are naturally permeable, without which there wouldn't be the transfer of enzymes through the gut walls for digestion and metabolism.

But the problem arises when they become excessively permeable, thereby causing a risk to the proper, smooth functioning of the digestive system. This condition is medically called leaky gut syndrome.

Multiple factors lead to a leaky gut, with diet and hazardous lifestyle habits being the major causes. The symptoms of a leaky gut can directly hamper the physiological and physical well-being of the individual. If one suffers from a leaky gut, it becomes imperative to fix this condition with medical treatment backed by lifestyle changes at the earliest opportunity.

10

BEYOND DIET

Contrary to popular belief, our gut constantly needs improvement and not just when we're battling gut disorders or recovering from an acute infection. Research has shown that about 10% of chronic conditions stem from genetic causes linked to the gut microbiome.

Owing to these factors, it becomes highly imperative to keep tabs on the functioning of the gut even when there are no apparent symptoms. Keep an eye out for other reactions in the rest of the body that can be attributed to poor gut health.

These symptoms include joint aches, acne-prone skin, anxiety and restlessness, loss of appetite, and so on. Beyond managing your diet and eating habits, here are

11 ways by which you can ensure the safety and smooth working of your gut.

All you need to do is use one or a few of these suggestions in your daily life while closely monitoring your diet intake and eating habits. Soon enough, you'll start witnessing the magic of good gut health in your system.

1. Check your stress levels:

Stress is one of the leading contributors to damaging physical health in all aspects. It increases your heart rate, induces palpitations, slows down metabolism, prevents smooth respiration, and can hinder the digestive process.

A hectic lifestyle combined with chronic stress only leads to loss of appetite. Loss of appetite, in turn, eventually translates into poor gut health. Therefore, practice calming and relaxing techniques like meditation, yoga, and art therapy to keep your stress levels under control.

Not only that, make it a point never to let stress dictate your appetite. Always consume a well-balanced diet and take all your meals in a timely fashion throughout the day to help you fight off stress better.

2. Avoid antibiotics:

Antibiotics are designed to get rid of the harmful bacteria in your gut to improve gut health. However, along with killing the harmful bacteria, the antibiotic medicines also attack the good bacteria and probiotics in the gut, weakening the gut microbiota further.

It eventually leads to low immunity and a compromised gut microbiome. Therefore, the best course of action is to avoid antibiotics at all costs until necessary. And even when you do have to consume them, make sure you complete the prescribed medicinal course to prevent the harmful bacteria from becoming drug-resistant over time.

3. Get moving:

Diet plays a huge role in determining the overall gut health of the individual, but the body also needs a little bit of exercise to help stay fit and toned. Working out a little bit each day stimulates blood flow and promotes a healthy, robust gut over time.

All you need to do is start slow and small. Stay steady with the minor changes in your schedule and build upon them gradually. Integrate physical activity into your daily schedule if you cannot dedicate specific hours to exercising each day.

Walk wherever possible, take the stairs when you can, take a brisk walk in your home office every hour, or walk your dog whenever you get the chance! Life gives you umpteen opportunities every day to stay active and fit. So go ahead and use them!

4. Drink enough water:

Staying hydrated is one of the main requirements of the gut. You can try all tactics to monitor your gut health, but your gut will suffer the most if your body is dehydrated.

Constipation, improper nutrient absorption, and difficulty in smooth bowel movements all occur due to dehydration. If there's a shortage of enough water in your system, the large intestine will suck out all water content from the food matter.

If this occurs frequently, it becomes difficult for the nitrogenous and toxic waste to be expelled quickly from the colon. Furthermore, being hydrated is imperative to regulate blood sugar, keep your mind fresh and active, and regulate your heart rate at all times. The effects of dehydration become quite visible over time, leading to dry and dull skin and overall weakened immunity.

5. Sleep:

The sleep hormone melatonin has an intimate connection with gut health. Sleep deprivation occurs when the production of melatonin is reduced in the system. This effect raises the levels of the hunger hormone, ghrelin, in the body while reducing the secretion of leptin, the hormone that suppresses hunger.

These converse actions of the hunger and sleep hormones compel your body to run on a regular circadian rhythm with both the digestive and the sleep cycles in sync.

We tend to overeat on the days that we are sleep-deprived. This occurs because of the converse relationship of both sets of hormones. Also, a well-rested body that has slept enough doesn't crave food as much as a sleep-deprived body.

6. Eat slowly:

One of the most basic rules of eating is to concentrate on the food on your plate. Keep away all distractions, work, gadgets, and essential discussions for later. Only light-hearted, casual talks are allowed when having meals.

Eat slowly, paying close attention to the smell, taste, and texture of the food on your plate and, eventually, in your mouth. Relish the flavors and be conscious of how your body is responding.

Moreover, eating slowly gives your body time to signal to you to stop eating as soon as the stomach is full. If you eat hastily or are distracted while eating, you'll surely miss these signs of fullness and end up overeating.

Overeating occasionally isn't so harmful, but a chronic habit of eating more than you need can lead to various disorders like high blood sugar, increased cholesterol levels, and obesity in the near future.

7. **Reduce gas:**

Accumulation of gases and acids in the gut leads to bloating and constipation. Hence, lay out your eating habits in such a way that there is little to no accumulation of gas in your system. You can employ some steps like:

- Eating slowly.
- Avoiding carbonated drinks.

- Reducing foods that cause heartburn.
- Holding in your bowel movements for longer than usual.

These habits listed are designed to reduce gas. Not following these guidelines can lead to gas buildup and, by consequence, an unhealthy gut.

8. Check for allergies:

Often, we fail to diagnose specific food allergies or food sensitivities that our bodies may be battling. There have been reports of people not being aware of their allergies until someone else points it out. In such cases, we can wrongly attribute the physical responses to poor gut health.

The solution is to have a quick health checkup to know about all your allergies, if any. You can then design your meal plans and dietary choices around your allergies. Taking this precaution will prevent your gut from suffering the health consequences of any accidental sensitivity or allergy.

9. Adopt a furry friend:

Having a pet around creates an indirect, profound impact on the gut microbiome. Recent research theories show that exposing young children to pets under controlled environments can help build strong immunity in the early childhood years.

The dirt on the pet's paws may seem like the worst idea for your baby, but it works like a charm to improve their immunity. This is true for adults as well. Get a furry friend and spend time with them to boost the diversity of your gut microbiome, thereby paving the way to more robust immunity.

10. Soak up vitamin D:

The early morning sun rays are an excellent source of vitamin D which is crucial to help you absorb calcium for your bones and teeth. Without enough vitamin D, there cannot be a healthy absorption of minerals like calcium, creating a deficiency in the body.

An absence of any nutrients in your system will create a direct impact on gut health. Hence, make it a point to soak up vitamin D early in the morning for a healthy start to the day.

11. Brush and floss teeth:

Plaque buildup around the teeth and the gums does have an impact on gut health. Any excess bacterial accumulation within the mouth also enters the gut through food.

Therefore, it is imperative to keep your oral hygiene in check to avoid the entry of any bacterial buildup inside the gut.

Regularly flossing the teeth, brushing at least twice a day, rinsing the entire mouth with an antibacterial mouthwash, and keeping your sugar intake in check are only a few ways by which you can ensure a hygienic mouth. Maintaining good oral hygiene prevents the entry of any harmful microbes into the gut.

QUICK RECAP

Diet and lifestyle habits are like the two oars of the same boat. One cannot work without the other. While diet and eating habits play a huge role in this regard, so do lifestyle habits. Working out, looking after your sleep cycle, and keeping stress levels in check are some of the most practical ways to ensure a healthy gut in addition to eating well.

AFTERWORD

The human body is miraculous in itself. It doesn't need constant attention to keep running in the best manner. The vital systems inside our body know their functions down to the core and are already performing to the best of their individual abilities and situations.

However, as responsible dwellers of this body, it is our foremost duty to provide our body with the best nourishment and lifestyle patterns to improve its performance as much as possible. Only when we strive for the betterment of our body can we ensure that it lasts long and well, houses our consciousness in the best way possible.

The core health of the body relies on how the gut performs. The function of the gastrointestinal tract largely determines the overall health of our body. Hence, it is our responsibility to give special care and attention to our gut so that it translates into better health for the whole body.

Looking after the gut comes in various forms. Here is a brief summary of some methods to help you:

- Eat well and right. Plenty of fiber, probiotics, prebiotics in your diet, please.
- Get enough sleep, watch your circadian rhythm closely.
- Cut down on junk food, processed foods, sugary meals, and fast food in your everyday life, if that's a norm you live by.
- Pay attention to oral hygiene. It influences our gut health more than we possibly know.
- Include vitamin and mineral supplements with the prior permission of your healthcare provider.

All you need to do is carry out the basic necessary steps in order to fulfill the needs of the gut, and leave the rest to your body to look after itself. Empowering our systems with the right steps is all that we need to go forward in the right direction to aid our good health.

REFERENCES

CHAPTER ONE:

1. Cheng, L. K., O'Grady, G., Du, P., Egbuji, J. U., Windsor, J. A., & Pullan, A.J. (2010, January). Gastrointestinal System. *WIREs Systems Biology and Medicine, 2*(1), 65–79. https://www.ncbi.nlm.nih.gov/pmc/articles/PMC4221587/

2. Merck Manuals Consumer Version. (2019, October). *Overview of the digestive system.* http://www.merckmanuals.com/home/digestive_disorders/biology_of_the_digestive_system/overview_of_the_digestive_system.html?qt=digestive&alt=sh

3. National Cancer Institute SEER Training Modules. (n.d.). *Introduction to the digestive system.* https://training.seer.cancer.gov/anatomy/digestive/

4. National Institute of Diabetes and Digestive and Kidney Diseases. (2017, December 30). *Your digestive system and how it works.* https://www.niddk.nih.gov/health-information/digestive-diseases/digestive-system-how-it-works

5. Patel, K. S., & Thavamani, A. (2021, March 1). *Physiology, peristalsis.* NCBI Bookshelf—StatPearls Publishing. https://www.ncbi.nlm.nih.gov/books/NBK556137/

6. A Review of 10 Years of Human Microbiome Research Activities at the US National Institutes of Health, Fiscal Years 2007–2016. (2019). *Microbiome, 7*(1). https://doi.org/10.1186/s40168-019-0620-y

7. Shreiner, A. B., Kao, J. Y., & Young, V. B. (2015, January). The Gut Microbiome in Health and in Disease. *Current Opinion in Gastroenterology, 31*(1), 69–75. https://doi.org/10.1097/MOG.0000000000000139

8. Svihus, B., & Itani, K. (2019, September). Intestinal Passage and Its Relation to Digestive Processes. *Journal of Applied Poultry Research, 28*(3), 546–555. https://www.sciencedirect.com/science/article/pii/S1056617119300583

CHAPTER TWO:

9. Bull, M. J., & Plummer, N. T. (2014). Part 1: The Human Gut Microbiome in Health and Disease. *Integrative Medicine (Encinitas, Calif.), 13*(6), 17–22. https://www.ncbi.nlm.nih.gov/pmc/articles/PMC4566439/

10. Cani, P. D. (2018). Human Gut Microbiome: Hopes, Threats and Promises. *Gut, 67*, 1716–1725. https://gut.bmj.com/content/67/9/1716

11. Durack, J., & Lynch, S. V. (2019). The Gut Microbiome: Relationships with Disease and Opportunities for Therapy. *Journal of Experimental Medicine, 216*(1), 20–40. https://doi.org/10.1084/jem.20180448

12. Goodrich, J. K., Waters, J. L., Poole, A. C., Sutter, J. L., Koren, O., Blekhman, R., Beaumont, M., Van Treuren, W., Knight, R., Bell, J. T., Spector, T. D., Clark, A. G., & Ley, R. E. Human Genetics Shape the Gut Microbiome. (2014, November). *Cell, 159*(4), 789–799. https://doi.org/10.1016/j.cell.2014.09.053

13. Heintz-Buschart, A., & Wilmes, P. (2017, November). Human Gut Microbiome: Function Matters. *Trends in Microbiology*, 26(7), 563–574. https://doi.org/10.1016/j.tim.2017.11.002

14. Microbiome research in general and business newspapers: How many microbiome articles are published and which study designs make the news the most? Andreu Prados-Bo, Gonzalo Casino, Published: April 9, 2021. https://doi.org/10.1371/journal.pone.0249835

15. Grace A. Ogunrinola, John O. Oyewale, Oyewumi O. Oshamika, Grace I. Olasehinde The Human Microbiome and Its Impacts on Health, International Journal of Microbiology, vol. 2020, Article ID 8045646, 7 pages, 2020. https://doi.org/10.1155/2020/8045646

16. Shreiner, A. B., Kao, J. Y., & Young, V. B. (2015, January). The Gut Microbiome in Health and in Disease. *Current Opinion in Gastroenterology, 31*(1), 69–75. https://doi.org/10.1097/MOG.0000000000000139

CHAPTER THREE:

17. Aoun, A., Darwish, F., & Hamod, N. (2020). The Influence of the Gut Microbiome on Obesity in Adults and the Role of Probiotics, Prebiotics, and Synbiotics for Weight Loss. Preventive nutrition and food science, 25(2), 113–123. https://doi.org/10.3746/pnf.2020.25.2.113

18. Bull, M. J., & Plummer, N. T. (2014). Part 1: The Human Gut Microbiome in Health and Disease. Integrative medicine (Encinitas, Calif.), 13(6), 17–22. https://www.ncbi.nlm.nih.gov/pmc/articles/PMC4566439/

19. Carabotti, M., Scirocco, A., Maselli, M. A., & Severi, C. (2015). The gut-brain axis: interactions between enteric microbiota, central and enteric nervous systems. Annals of gastroenterology, 28(2), 203–209. https://www.ncbi.nlm.nih.gov/pmc/articles/PMC4367209/

20. Chandran, Suhas & Manohari, Shroff & Raman, Vijaya. (2019). The gut-brain connection: A qualitative review of the conceptualisation and implications of the gut-brain-microbiome axis. Telangana Journal of Psychiatry. 5. 94. 10.18231/j.tjp.2019.022. https://www.researchgate.net/publication/337740900_The_gut-brain_connection_A_qualitative_review_of_the_conceptualisation_and_implications_of_the_gut-brain-microbiome_axis

21. Maria Carlota Dao, Amandine Everard, Karine Clément, Patrice D. Cani. Losing weight for a better health: Role for the gut microbiota, Clinical Nutrition Experimental, Volume 6, 2016, Pages 39–58, ISSN 2352–9393. https://doi.org/10.1016/j.yclnex.2015.12.001

22. Davis C. D. (2016). The Gut Microbiome and Its Role in Obesity. Nutrition today, 51(4), 167–174. https://doi.org/10.1097/NT.0000000000000167

23. De Pessemier, B., Grine, L., Debaere, M., Maes, A., Paetzold, B., & Callewaert, C. (2021). Gut-Skin Axis: Current Knowledge of the Interrelationship between Microbial Dysbiosis and Skin Conditions. Microorganisms, 9(2), 353. https://doi.org/10.3390/microorganisms9020353

24. A psychology of the human brain-gut-microbiome axis; Andrew P. Allen, Timothy G. Dinan, Gerard Clarke, John F. Cryan, 18 April 2017 https://doi.org/10.1111/spc3.12309

25. Salem, I., Ramser, A., Isham, N., & Ghannoum, M. A. (2018). The Gut Microbiome as a Major Regulator of the Gut-Skin Axis. Frontiers in microbiology, 9, 1459. https://doi.org/10.3389/fmicb.2018.01459

26. Targeting the gut-skin axis—Probiotics as new tools for skin disorder management? Magdolna Szántó, Anikó Dózsa, Dóra Antal, Kornélia Szabó, Lajos Kemény, Péter Bai, First published: 06 August 2019. https://doi.org/10.1111/exd.14016

CHAPTER FOUR:

27. M. Choct (2009) Managing gut health through nutrition, British Poultry Science, 50:1, 9–15, DOI: 10.1080/00071660802538632. https://www.

tandfonline.com/doi/full/10.1080/
00071660802538632?scroll=top&needAccess=true

28. De Luca, F., & Shoenfeld, Y. The microbiome in autoimmune diseases. *Clinical & Experimental Immunology*. 2019 Jan;195(1):74–85. doi: 10.1111/cei.13158. PMID: 29920643; PMCID: PMC6300652. https://pubmed.ncbi.nlm.nih.gov/29920643/

29. Lobionda, S., Sittipo, P., Kwon, H. Y., & Lee, Y. K. (2019). The Role of Gut Microbiota in Intestinal Inflammation with Respect to Diet and Extrinsic Stressors. Microorganisms, 7(8), 271. https://doi.org/10.3390/microorganisms7080271

30. Quigley E. M. (2013). Gut bacteria in health and disease. Gastroenterology & hepatology, 9(9), 560–569. https://www.ncbi.nlm.nih.gov/pmc/articles/PMC3983973/

31. The Relationship Between Gut Microbiota and Inflammatory Diseases: The Role of Macrophages, Ji Wang, Wei-Dong Chen, and Yan-Dong Wang, *Frontiers in Microbiology*, 09 June 2020. https://doi.org/10.3389/fmicb.2020.01065

32. Role of the gut microbiota in nutrition and health, (Published 13 June 2018), BMJ 2018; 361. doi: https://doi.org/10.1136/bmj.k2179

33. Saha L. (2014). Irritable bowel syndrome: Pathogenesis, diagnosis, treatment, and evidence-based medicine. World journal of gastroenterology, 20(22), 6759–6773. https://doi.org/10.3748/wjg.v20.i22.6759

34. Vahedi, H., Ansari, R., Mir-Nasseri, M., & Jafari, E. (2010). Irritable bowel syndrome: A review article. Middle East journal of digestive diseases, 2(2), 66–77. https://www.ncbi.nlm.nih.gov/pmc/articles/PMC4154827/

35. Xu, H., Liu, M., Cao, J., Li, X., Fan, D., Xia, Y., Lu, X., Li, J., Ju, D., & Zhao, H. (2019). The Dynamic Interplay between the Gut Microbiota and Autoimmune Diseases. Journal of immunology research, 2019, 7546047. https://doi.org/10.1155/2019/7546047

36. Zhang, Y. J., Li, S., Gan, R. Y., Zhou, T., Xu, D. P., & Li, H. B. (2015). Impacts of gut bacteria on human health and diseases. International journal of molecular sciences, 16(4), 7493–7519. https://doi.org/10.3390/ijms16047493

CHAPTER FIVE:

37. Abuajah, C. I., Ogbonna, A. C., & Osuji, C. M. (2015). Functional components and medicinal properties of food: A review. Journal of Food Science and

Technology, 52, 2522–2529. https://doi.org/10.1007/s13197-014-1396-5

38. Al-Sheraji, S. H., Ismail, A., Manap, M. Y., Mustafa, S., Yusof, R. M., & Hassan, F. A. (2013). Prebiotics as functional foods: A review. Journal of Functional Foods, 5, 1542–1553. https://doi.org/10.1016/j.jff.2013.08.009

39. Amy M. Brownawell, Wim Caers, Glenn R. Gibson, Cyril W. C. Kendall, Kara D. Lewis, Yehuda Ringel, Joanne L. Slavin, Prebiotics and the Health Benefits of Fiber: Current Regulatory Status, Future Research, and Goals, The Journal of Nutrition, Volume 142, Issue 5, May 2012, Pages 962–974. https://doi.org/10.3945/jn.112.158147

40. Carlson, J. L., Erickson, J. M., Lloyd, B. B., & Slavin, J. L. (2018). Health Effects and Sources of Prebiotic Dietary Fiber. Current developments in nutrition, 2(3), nzy005. https://doi.org/10.1093/cdn/nzy005

41. Davani-Davari, D., Negahdaripour, M., Karimzadeh, I., Seifan, M., Mohkam, M., Masoumi, S. J., Berenjian, A., & Ghasemi, Y. (2019). Prebiotics: Definition, Types, Sources, 42. Mechanisms, and Clinical Applications. Foods (Basel, Switzerland), 8(3), 92. https://doi.org/10.3390/foods8030092

43. Effectiveness of probiotics, prebiotics, and prebiotic-like components in common functional foods; Mengfei Peng, Zajeba Tabashsum, Mary Anderson, Andy Truong, Ashley K. Houser, Joselyn Padilla, Ahlam Akmel, Jacob Bhatti, Shaik O. Rahaman, Debabrata Biswa. https://doi.org/10.1111/1541-4337.12565

44. Roberfroid M, Gibson GR, Hoyles L, McCartney AL, Rastall R, Rowland I, Wolvers D, Watzl B, Szajewska H, Stahl B, Guarner F, Respondek F, Whelan K, Coxam V, Davicco MJ, Léotoing L, Wittrant Y, Delzenne NM, Cani PD, Neyrinck AM, Meheust A. Prebiotic effects: metabolic and health benefits. *The British Journal of Nutrition*. 2010 Aug;104 Suppl 2:S1-63. doi: 10.1017/S0007114510003363. PMID: 20920376. https://pubmed.ncbi.nlm.nih.gov/20920376/

45. Slavin J. Fiber and Prebiotics: Mechanisms and Health Benefits. Nutrients. 2013; 5(4):1417–1435. https://doi.org/10.3390/nu5041417

46. Thammarutwasik, Paiboon & Hongpattarakere, Tipparat & Chantachum, Suphitchaya & Kijroongrojana, Kongkarn & Itharat, Arunporn & Reanmongkol, Wantana & Tewtrakul, Supinya & Ooraikul, Buncha. (2009). Prebiotics - A Review. Songklanakarin Journal of Science and Technology. 31. 401–408. https://www.researchgate.net/publication/279902625_Prebiotics_-_A_Review

CHAPTER SIX:

47. Effects of probiotics on gut microbiota: mechanisms of intestinal immunomodulation and neuromodulation, Peera Hemarajata and James Versalovic https://www.ncbi.nlm.nih.gov/pmc/articles/PMC3539293/

48. Ford AC, Harris LA, Lacy BE, et al. Systematic review with meta-analysis: the efficacy of prebiotics, probiotics, synbiotics and antibiotics in irritable bowel syndrome. Alimentary Pharmacology & Therapeutics. 2018;48(10):1044–1060. https://pubmed.ncbi.nlm.nih.gov/30294792/

49. Maria Kechagia, Dimitrios Basoulis, Stavroula Konstantopoulou, Dimitra Dimitriadi, Konstantina Gyftopoulou, Nikoletta Skarmoutsou, Eleni Maria Fakiri. Health Benefits of Probiotics: A Review. International Scholarly Research Notices, vol. 2013, Article ID 481651, 7 pages, 2013. https://doi.org/10.5402/2013/481651

50. Kechagia, Maria & Basoulis, Dimitrios & Konstantopoulou, Stavroula & Dimitriadi, Dimitra & Gyftopoulou, Konstantina & Skarmoutsou, Nikoletta & Fakiri, Eleni. (2013). Health Benefits of Probiotics: A Review. ISRN Nutrition. 2013. 10.5402/2013/481651. https://www.researchgate.net/

publication/258405079_Health_Benefits_of_Probiotics_A_Review

51. Health Benefits of Probiotics: A Review; Maria Kechagia, Dimitrios Basoulis, Stavroula Konstantopoulou, Dimitra Dimitriadi, Konstantina Gyftopoulou, Nikoletta Skarmoutsou, and Eleni Maria Fakiri. https://www.ncbi.nlm.nih.gov/pmc/articles/PMC4045285/

52. Effects of Probiotics, Prebiotics, and Synbiotics on Human Health. Paulina Markowiak and Katarzyna Śliżewska. https://www.ncbi.nlm.nih.gov/pmc/articles/PMC5622781/

53. Seerengeraj, Vijayaram. (2018). Probiotics: The Marvelous Factor and Health Benefits. Biomedical and Biotechnology Research Journal (BBRJ). 2. 1-8. 10.4103/bbrj.bbrj_87_17. https://www.researchgate.net/publication/323639630_Probiotics_The_Marvelous_Factor_and_Health_Benefits

54. Probiotics in Food Systems: Significance and Emerging Strategies Towards Improved Viability and Delivery of Enhanced Beneficial Value; Antonia Terpou, Aikaterini Papadaki, Iliada K. Lappa, Vasiliki Kachrimanidou, Loulouda A. Bosnea, and Nikolaos

Kopsahelis. https://www.ncbi.nlm.nih.gov/pmc/articles/PMC6683253/

55. Zhao, Wenbin & Liu, Yuheng & Latta, Maria & Ma, Wantong & Wu, Zhengrong & Chen, Peng. (2019). Probiotics database: a potential source of fermented foods. International Journal of Food Properties. 22. 197–216. 10.1080/10942912.2019.1579737. https://www.researchgate.net/publication/331255481_Probiotics_database_a_potential_source_of_fermented_foods

56. Probiotics database: a potential source of fermented foods; Wenbin Zhao, Yuheng Liu, Maria Latta, Wantong Ma, Zhengrong Wu &Peng Chen, Pages 198–217. https://www.tandfonline.com/doi/full/10.1080/10942912.2019.1579737

CHAPTER SEVEN:

57. Kembra Albracht-Schulte, Tariful Islam, Paige Johnson, Naima Moustaid-Moussa, Systematic Review of Beef Protein Effects on Gut Microbiota: Implications for Health, Advances in Nutrition, Volume 12, Issue 1, January 2021, Pages 102–114, https://doi.org/10.1093/advances/nmaa085

58. Baojun, X., Christudas, S., & Devaraj, R. (2020). Different impacts of plant proteins and animal proteins on human health through altering gut microbiota. Functional Foods in Health and Disease. 10. 10.31989/ffhd.v10i5.699. https://www.researchgate.net/publication/341583206_Different_impacts_of_plant_proteins_and_animal_proteins_on_human_health_through_altering_gut_microbiotaant_proteins_and_animal_proteins_on_human_health_through_altering_gut_microbiota

59. Conlon, M. A., & Bird, A. R. (2014). The impact of diet and lifestyle on gut microbiota and human health. Nutrients, 7(1), 17–44. https://doi.org/10.3390/nu7010017

60. Journal of Gastroenterology and Hepatology, Processed food affects the gut microbiota: The revolution has started, Michael A Kamm MD, PhD, First published: 21 January 2020 https://doi.org/10.1111/jgh.14976

61. Kruis, W., Forstmaier, G., Scheurlen, C., & Stellaard, F. (1991). Effect of diets low and high in refined sugars on gut transit, bile acid metabolism, and bacterial fermentation. Gut, 32(4), 367–371. https://doi.org/10.1136/gut.32.4.367

62. Madsen, L., Myrmel, L. S., Fjære, E., Liaset, B., & Kristiansen, K. (2017). Links between Dietary Protein Sources, the Gut Microbiota, and Obesity. Frontiers in physiology, 8, 1047. https://doi.org/10.3389/fphys.2017.01047

63. Miclotte L, Van de Wiele T. Food processing, gut microbiota and the globesity problem. Crit Rev Food Sci Nutr. 2020;60(11):1769-1782. doi: 10.1080/10408398.2019.1596878. Epub 2019 Apr 4. PMID: 30945554. https://pubmed.ncbi.nlm.nih.gov/30945554/

64. Shi Z. (2019). Gut Microbiota: An Important Link between Western Diet and Chronic Diseases. Nutrients, 11(10), 2287. https://doi.org/10.3390/nu11102287

65. Singh, R. K., Chang, H. W., Yan, D., Lee, K. M., Ucmak, D., Wong, K., Abrouk, M., Farahnik, B., Nakamura, M., Zhu, T. H., Bhutani, T., & Liao, W. (2017). Influence of diet on the gut microbiome and implications for human health. Journal of translational medicine, 15(1), 73. https://doi.org/10.1186/s12967-017-1175-y

66. Satokari R. (2020). High Intake of Sugar and the Balance between Pro- and Anti-Inflammatory Gut Bacteria. Nutrients, 12(5), 1348. https://doi.org/10.3390/nu12051348

CHAPTER EIGHT:

67. Blumberg, J. B., Bailey, R. L., Sesso, H. D., & Ulrich, C. M. (2018). The Evolving Role of Multivitamin/Multimineral Supplement Use among Adults in the Age of Personalized Nutrition. Nutrients, 10(2), 248. https://doi.org/10.3390/nu10020248

68. Hu FB: Plant-based foods and prevention of cardiovascular disease: an overview. *The American Journal of Cinical Nutrition*. 2003, 78: 544S-551S.

69. Ward, E. Addressing nutritional gaps with multivitamin and mineral supplements. *Nutrition Journal,* 13, 72 (2014). https://doi.org/10.1186/1475-2891-13-72

70. Yang, Q., Liang, Q., Balakrishnan, B., Belobrajdic, D. P., Feng, Q. J., & Zhang, W. (2020). Role of Dietary Nutrients in the Modulation of Gut Microbiota: A Narrative Review. Nutrients, 12(2), 381. https://doi.org/10.3390/nu12020381

71. Health effects of vitamin and mineral supplements, BMJ 2020; 369 doi: https://doi.org/10.1136/bmj.m2511

CHAPTER NINE:

72. Hans-Joachim Anders, Kirstin Andersen, Bärbel Stecher, The intestinal microbiota, a leaky gut, and abnormal immunity in kidney disease, Kidney International, Volume 83, Issue 6, 2013, Pages 1010–1016, ISSN 0085-2538, https://doi.org/10.1038/ki.2012.440.

73. Camilleri M. (2019). Leaky gut: mechanisms, measurement and clinical implications in humans. Gut, 68(8), 1516–1526. https://doi.org/10.1136/gutjnl-2019-318427

74. Fasano, A. Leaky Gut and Autoimmune Diseases. *Clinical Reviews in Allergy & Immunology,* 42, 71–78 (2012). https://doi.org/10.1007/s12016-011-8291-x

75. Fasano A. (2020). All disease begins in the (leaky) gut: role of zonulin-mediated gut permeability in the pathogenesis of some chronic inflammatory diseases. F1000Research, 9, F1000 Faculty Rev-69. https://doi.org/10.12688/f1000research.20510.1

76. Fasano A. All disease begins in the (leaky) gut: role of zonulin-mediated gut permeability in the pathogenesis of some chronic inflammatory diseases [version 1; peer review: 3 approved]. F1000Research 2020,

9(F1000 Faculty Rev):69 https://doi.org/10.12688/f1000research.20510.1

77. Mu, Q., Kirby, J., Reilly, C. M., & Luo, X. M. (2017). Leaky Gut as a Danger Signal for Autoimmune Diseases. Frontiers in immunology, 8, 598. https://doi.org/10.3389/fimmu.2017.00598

78. Mu Qinghui, Kirby Jay, Reilly Christopher M., Luo Xin M, Leaky Gut as a Danger Signal for Autoimmune Diseases, Frontiers in Immunology, Volume 8, 2017 https://www.frontiersin.org/article/10.3389/fimmu.2017.00598

79. Obrenovich MEM. Leaky Gut, Leaky Brain? Microorganisms. 2018; 6(4):107. https://doi.org/10.3390/microorganisms6040107

80. Paray BA, Albeshr MF, Jan AT, Rather IA. Leaky Gut and Autoimmunity: An Intricate Balance in Individuals Health and the Diseased State. International Journal of Molecular Sciences. 2020; 21(24):9770. https://doi.org/10.3390/ijms21249770

81. Kinashi Yusuke, Hase Koji, Partners in Leaky Gut Syndrome: Intestinal Dysbiosis and Autoimmunity, Frontiers in Immunology, Volume 12, 2021, DOI=10.3389/fimmu.2021.673708, ISSN 1664-3224 https://www.frontiersin.org/article/10.3389/fimmu.2021.673708

CHAPTER TEN:

82. David, L. A., Maurice, C. F., Carmody, R. N., Gootenberg, D. B., Button, J. E., Wolfe, B. E., Ling, A. V., Devlin, A. S., Varma, Y., Fischbach, M. A., Biddinger, S. B., Dutton, R. J., & Turnbaugh, P. J. (2014). Diet rapidly and reproducibly alters the human gut microbiome. Nature, 505(7484), 559–563. https://doi.org/10.1038/nature12820

83. Galley, J. D., Nelson, M. C., Yu, Z., Dowd, S. E., Walter, J., Kumar, P. S., Lyte, M., & Bailey, M. T. (2014). Exposure to a social stressor disrupts the community structure of the colonic mucosa-associated microbiota. BMC microbiology, 14, 189. https://doi.org/10.1186/1471-2180-14-189

84. Hasler W. L. (2006). Gas and Bloating. Gastroenterology & hepatology, 2(9), 654–662. https://www.ncbi.nlm.nih.gov/pmc/articles/PMC5350578/

85. Hills, R. D., Jr, Pontefract, B. A., Mishcon, H. R., Black, C. A., Sutton, S. C., & Theberge, C. R. (2019). Gut Microbiome: Profound Implications for Diet and Disease. Nutrients, 11(7), 1613. https://doi.org/10.3390/nu11071613

86. Magnusson KR, Hauck L, Jeffrey BM, Elias V, Humphrey A, Nath R, Perrone A, Bermudez LE. Relationships between diet-related changes in the gut microbiome and cognitive flexibility. Neuroscience. 2015 Aug 6;300:128-40. doi: 10.1016/j.neuroscience.2015.05.016. Epub 2015 May 14. PMID: 25982560. https://pubmed.ncbi.nlm.nih.gov/25982560/

87. Olsen, I., & Yamazaki, K. (2019). Can oral bacteria affect the microbiome of the gut? Journal of oral microbiology, 11(1), 1586422. https://doi.org/10.1080/20002297.2019.1586422

88. Pascal, M., Perez-Gordo, M., Caballero, T., Escribese, M. M., Lopez Longo, M. N., Luengo, O., Manso, L., Matheu, V., Seoane, E., Zamorano, M., Labrador, M., & Mayorga, C. (2018). Microbiome and Allergic Diseases. Frontiers in immunology, 9, 1584. https://doi.org/10.3389/fimmu.2018.01584

89. Petriz, B. A., Castro, A. P., Almeida, J. A., Gomes, C. P., Fernandes, G. R., Kruger, R. H., Pereira, R. W., & Franco, O. L. (2014). Exercise induction of gut microbiota modifications in obese, non-obese and hypertensive rats. BMC genomics, 15(1), 511. https://doi.org/10.1186/1471-2164-15-511

90. Suez J, Korem T, Zeevi D, Zilberman-Schapira G, Thaiss CA, Maza O, Israeli D, Zmora N, Gilad S, Weinberger A, Kuperman Y, Harmelin A, Kolodkin-Gal I,

Shapiro H, Halpern Z, Segal E, Elinav E. Artificial sweeteners induce glucose intolerance by altering the gut microbiota. Nature. 2014 Oct 9;514(7521):181-6. doi: 10.1038/nature13793. Epub 2014 Sep 17. PMID: 25231862. https://pubmed.ncbi.nlm.nih.gov/25231862/

91. Voigt, R. M., Forsyth, C. B., Green, S. J., Mutlu, E., Engen, P., Vitaterna, M. H., Turek, F. W., & Keshavarzian, A. (2014). Circadian disorganization alters intestinal microbiota. *PLOS ONE*, 9(5), e97500. https://doi.org/10.1371/journal.pone.0097500

Printed in Poland
by Amazon Fulfillment
Poland Sp. z o.o., Wrocław